ABC's of Reflexology

ABC's of Reflexology

Benita and Jim Babeckis

Published for:
TRANZFORMATIONS
Oro Valley, Az. 85704

Email: Tranzform@Comcast.net
Website: http:// Tranzformations.net

Published for Tranzformations
8571 N. Calle Tioga
Oro Valley, Arizona 85704

ISBN No. 978-1500625900

First Published September, 2014
Text and diagrams updated 2016

Manufactured in the United States of America

Contents

Contents

Diagrams

Preface

The material being presented here was first assembled and organized as a class to be presented live to those who wanted to learn Reflexology as a career. This was in 2010. In 2014 the material was revised into its present form and is being presented as this book. Chapter XI is a remnant of this. Other traces may still exist as well.

Reflexology is the practice of applying pressure (to stimulate and activate the nerves) in the feet and hands. Reflexology is based on a system of zones, that reflects an image of the body on the feet and hands which in turn effects the physical changes made in the body.

Reflexology is a popular method of detecting and addressing any possible ailments, illnesses, or diseases the body may be experiencing.

In ancient times this method was used to ensure that any possible health problems in the body were caught before they progressed to where they would be more difficult to treat.

Chapter I

Grounding and Centering for Therapists

> Because our mental energies are always in flux it is important to "check in" with our bodies (both physical and energy bodies) routinely to adjust and center ourselves.

The process of relaxing and making yourself receptive and present for any activity is called grounding and centering. It is a foundational tool of many traditions and therapies.

Grounding literally means visualizing yourself connected to the earth. Once you are grounded, you then visualize yourself centered in the present instead of constantly thinking of the past or the future. The reasoning behind this is that you do not want to start a session in your everyday state of mind with all of your stresses and thoughts everywhere but on the client in front of you.

It is best to let your daily disturbances fall by the wayside even if it is only for the length of your intended session. With a clear mind you will be better able to work for your client and both of you will benefit.

If you find yourself stubbing your toes or bumping into things, you are not in balance. If you are experiencing mental confusion or are all over the place emotionally, a centering visualization can help return you to calm and better focus.

Centering

Close your eyes, and place your feet firmly on the ground or floor. Gather all your energy into a warm, glowing ball in the center of your body. (just below the Navel). Find a center point in yourself and feel it there, steady and calm., maintain this as long as you need to, until you feel calm and relaxed.

To be ungrounded means our thoughts are not in the body. It means you are upset, angry, spacey, frustrated, or emotional in some form or another. You are not experiencing the now. Typically, when we are ungrounded, we are thinking about something else besides what we are doing or being right now. It's usually experienced in a seemingly negative way, but not always. Sometimes we can just not be here - our soul is off somewhere else.

Think about traffic. How many people are driving around every day thinking about something else and not about their driving? Probably most drivers. This is why we have so many accidents. People are not paying attention to what they are doing. They are not grounded.

Grounding

Center yourself first. Grounding begins with the breath. Breathe deeply. Try this: clench your stomach, tighten your muscles, breath up high in your chest. How do you begin to feel? (People often say, "anxious," "Tense," "Panicky.") Now relax your stomach, let your breath drop down into your belly, into your toes as your belly expands. Do you start to feel different? For some of you, this might be hard to do. At first it might seem unnatural. Put your hand on your belly, breathe so that your belly pushes your hand out. Practice this, sometimes you need time before you can do it easily and naturally.

As you breathe in, feel the clean, fresh air filling your lungs, filling your Self. As you breathe slowly out, feel the worries and problems of your everyday life, your problems slipping away, through your feet into the Earth. Now imagine yourself slowly putting down roots, small at first, getting thicker, through your feet and your hands. Feel those roots get thicker as they go down through layers of soil and rock, pushing deep into the Earth Mother's body.

Imagine the water table under all those layers of earth, and when your roots reach the water, draw the cool, fresh energy of the Earth up to your core and merge with it - the Earth energy is a deep well, and you are drawing it into yourself, through your chakras, up your spine and through the top of your head. Feel the Earth energy fill you, rise through you like refreshing water, and feel it flow through your Center, constantly providing both new energy and a route for negative and unhealthy energy to flow away, carried by the Earth Power back to the depths of the living well to be cleansed and made useful again.

As the energy flows through the top of your head, feel it branch out, spreading like the arms of a tree. Feel it grow to the sky, into the stars, and touch the universal source pulsing overhead. As it pulses, draw it down through your branches, down through those arms and into your center, to connect with your Core, to join there in union and balance with the strength of the Earth. Feel the cool breezes of the source invigorate and cleanse you, bringing inspiration and joy from the vast Universe into your Center.

Now you are connected to Mother Earth, and the universe; feel them join together in a balance in your Center, and in your Self.

You are grounded now in all things, and may journey deeper into other realms; this is the beginning of a meditative state, the state in which the mind is ready for whatever comes.

The purpose of being grounded and centered is to make you present, truly present, "in" the moment.

When you are present, you can think clearly and interact with your surroundings, instead of reacting. You cannot control the future; you cannot control the past. But "in" the moment, you can do whatever you set your mind to do and by thinking clearly, being grounded and centered, whatever is needful will appear.

Grounding helps with maintaining a balance of our physical and spiritual bodies. As a healer, we have learned that being energetically grounded allows us to be better equipped in facilitating healing for clients and also to create and maintain wellness in our own life.

Now come back to stillness. As you breathe, feel where it is in your body this grounded place seems to live, and touch that place. Can you find an image for this grounded state?

A word or phrase you can say? When you use these three together, touch, image, and phrase, you create an anchor to help you ground quickly in any situation. Try it -- use it.

Now relax. How did that go for you all? What did you notice?

Remember, the more you practice grounding, the more automatic it becomes. If you take even a few minutes a day to practice, you'll not only have better energy in your daily life, you'll be able to ground quickly and instantly when you're in a tense situation.

Grounding Exercise: Body Scan

Bring your thoughts from busy mental chatter downward by focusing on your feet. Don't rush this process. Take your time moving from each part of your body. Also, you don't need to touch yourself, just allow your mind to switch focus from wherever it is. Begin with your feet and move upwards.

Notice the soles of your feet, your toes, in-between your toes, the top of your feet, the back of your ankle.

Do they feel hot? or cold? Do they hurt? Are they numb? Do you feel your blood circulating through them? Are they feeling tired?

Don't judge how they feel - just notice how they feel. Wiggle your toes. How does that feel?

Once you have a made a strong connection with your feet you may then move your attention upwards to your ankle... then switch focus to your lower legs, onto your knee caps, behind your knees, your thighs, and so on.

How can getting grounded Help me?

To become fully alive, we need to step out of our head, and dip our whole selves into the body, its senses, its feelings, the world, and the waters of life. We need to be grounded. Being grounded is fundamental to well-being and a balanced life. Grounding alleviates anxiety and panic. Grounding is recognized as an important component of any effort to remedy stress, anxiety, or panic attacks, because grounding directs the energy and awareness back into the body thereby helping to manage stress, catastrophic thinking, and panic. Being grounded calms the scattered daytime living and calms the scattered nighttime mind. Grounding clears the mind's film of thought, releasing us to engage a more vital and fulfilling life in relation to our bodies, feelings, and others.

The Personal Cost of Being Ungrounded

Do you have anxiety or panic attacks? Do you feel scattered, spacey, living too much in your head... or out of touch with your self and life? Most likely you're ungrounded! When we are not grounded, we live in the mind and intellect, out of touch with our bodies, feelings, and the world. It's as if we're living through a film of thought that separates us from others and life. We refuse life's invitation to become immersed in a world of sensory aliveness, immediacy, and aliveness..

When we are ungrounded, our energy is concentrated more in our heads. Sometimes we experience this as being spaced out, floating, living as if in a dream, absent-minded, klutzy, unaware of our bodies.

Sometimes we experience this 'spaciness' as even being unaware of our legs and feet or simply feeling numb to life below the neckline. We live from within the tower of the mind content to spend our lives in fantasy or other unbalanced intellectual pursuits. We'd prefer to read a book about love, rather than fall in love.

Sometimes feelings of stress, anxiety, or panic will lead to being ungrounded. And vice versa... being ungrounded can bring panic, anxiety, and stress.

We feel harried, scattered, 'running around like a chicken with its head cut off.' We can't slow down our thoughts. Our bodies are always on the move. We suffer from insomnia, our thoughts being ceaselessly on the move too.

All of these are signs that something is wrong.

An ungrounded life is a life whose mind and heart and body are not integrated. This lack of integration results in an imbalance of energy causing the bulk of the energy to be centered in the head. This can result in a seemingly endless mental chatter. We can't think straight. Or, we experience life as if we only were a (dissociated) head, having no or limited awareness of feelings and bodily sensations. Our awareness is centered in the head, rather than distributed throughout our body.

If you are unhappy with being ungrounded, you can do something about it! Getting grounded is a skill which you can develop, and make a way of life.

* * *

Notes

Chapter II

Introduction and Vocabulary

The primary purpose of this course is to give you an opportunity to learn and begin the practice of Reflexology.

On Being a Professional

The word profession has many meanings. According to the Merriam-Webster Collegiate Dictionary (2000), a profession is:
1. A calling requiring specialized knowledge, usually obtained by academic preparation
2. A principal calling, vocation or employment
3. The whole body of persons engaged in a calling.

In your opinion, what does it mean to be a "professional"? In our society, two of the concepts that distinguish professionals from nonprofessionals are *accountability* and *liability*. To be accountable means to be subject to giving an account or an explanation of one's actions.

To be "liable" means to be responsible and obligated according to law or equity. The term "professional liability" means the obligation of the professional to pay for damages resulting from his or her acts during contact with clients (Taber's, 1998) (see note at end of Chapter).

Another important hallmark of being a professional is the understanding and application of theory to the work. The word "theory" has several meanings, but the ones most applicable to this discussion are:

1. the general or abstract principles of a body of fact, science or art, as in "music theory" *

2. a belief, policy or procedure proposed or followed as the basis of action, as in "her method is based on the theory* that all children want to learn"

3. an ideal or hypothetical set of facts, principles or circumstances, used in a phrase, as in "in theory, we advocate freedom"

4. a plausible or scientifically acceptable general principle or body of principles offered to explain phenomena, as in "wave theory of light" (Merriam Webster, 2000)

5. a speculation, supposition or assumption based on certain evidence or observations, but lacking in scientific proof (Taber's, 1998)

* A synonym for "theory" is hypothesis.

When a theory becomes generally accepted and firmly established, it becomes a doctrine or a fundamental principle. Since humans first began to think and reflect, they have developed theories about what causes health, illness and healing, and how we should interact with those phenomena. Today there are thousands of theories based on the values, perspectives and experiences of thousands of groups of people.

The development of a professional theory starts with examining one's own personal theories, perspectives, experiences and values and extends to the theories that are accepted and approved by one's professional group or subgroup. What are your personal theories? What parts are congruent with each other, and what parts are in conflict? What parts of your theories are congruent with the dominant theories in your work or study groups? What parts are different? Where do you go to learn more and/or develop your theories? How do you apply them in daily life? How do you test them? These are a few of the central issues each of us face and respond to during our professional growth.

When a group of people want to establish themselves as professionals, one of the first things they do is define their work, or *practice*.

Taber's (1998) defines "practice" in relation to the health care professions as "the use of knowledge and skill to provide a service in the prevention, diagnosis and treatment of illness, and the maintenance of health." For example, a short definition of nursing practice is "the diagnosis and treatment of human responses to actual or potential health problems." A short definition of massage therapy is "the systematic therapeutic manipulation of the body's soft tissues by a specially trained therapist."

These short definitions are only starting points. Each profession eventually establishes, through arduous member discussion, a "Standards of Practice" statement. A "standard" is something established by authority, custom or general consent as a model or example. Therefore, Standards of Practice are the baseline criteria for acceptable practice. Standards of Practice serve several functions.
They:
- inform new members about the group's expectations
- inform the public, other professionals, businesses and regulatory agencies about the responsibilities they can expect from the group.

Another equally important step toward professionalism is the development of a Code of Ethics.

Based on the concepts of professionalism, body-centered therapists have an ethical and legal responsibility not to harm their clients. *Ethics* are a set of moral principles or values. A Code of Ethics is a collection of rules, regulations and/or specifications for governing conduct. Each professional group creates its own Code of Ethics to define what actions are good and bad, and where moral duty and obligation fall.

Professional Vocabulary

Accountability: to be subject to giving an account or an explanation of one's actions.

Acute: sharp, severe, as in *acute pain;* having a rapid onset, severe symptoms and a short course.

Aging: maturing; progressive changes related to the passage of time.

Assessment: the collection and interpretation of information provided by the client, any referring health professionals and your own observation .

Biomedical: modem medicine with application of the natural sciences.

Body/mind: the whole mental, physical, emotional, spiritual, social, environmental and energetic human being.

Body-centered therapy: any therapy that focuses its theory, knowledge and practice on achieving improved physiological outcomes, including massage therapy, bodywork, nursing, therapeutic movement, yoga instruction, personal training and others.

Boundary: a limit; may be in physical, emotional, financial or any other area; defines what will and will not occur between the therapist and client.

CAM: complementary/alternative medicine; an emerging set of diverse therapies in the U.S., having multi-cultural origins, in which two major principles are: respect for the client's body and values and the promotion and empowerment of health.

Chronic: of long duration; showing a slow progression.

Client goal: what the client wants from body-centered therapy.

Code of Ethics: a collection of rules, regulations and/or specifications for governing conduct.

Collaborate: cooperate or work jointly with others.

Confidentiality: right of each person to his or her privacy, including personal information obtained from or about a client.

Consent: the granting of permission by one person for an act to be carried out by another.

Contraindication: a persuasive reason to avoid a therapeutic action under consideration.

Counter transference: the projection by a therapist of feelings, needs or issues onto a client, instead of recognizing them as his or her own.

Critical thinking: attempting to think clearly, accurately and fairly while evaluating the reasons for accepting a belief or taking an action; in contrast to mere disagreement, critical thinking is useful for understanding and evaluating the support given for a point of view.

Diagnosis: the naming of a condition or problem.

Disability: a limited function in any aspect of the body/mind; some disabilities are visible and some are "invisible."

Disease: literally means a lack of ease and can include any group of symptoms distinct from normal health conditions; any impaired performance of a vital function, or any suffering that mayor may not arise from pathological changes.

Dual relationship: an alliance between the therapist and client that is outside, the usually contracted roles, e.g., social, romantic, business, familial, etc.

Effleurage: a gliding stroke in massage therapy; usually follows the direction of the underlying muscle fibers.

Energy field: a fundamental unit of the living and the nonliving; a unifying concept signifying the dynamic nature of infinite continuous motion and interconnectedness.

Ethics: discipline dealing with what is good and bad and with moral duty and obligation; principles or values.

Etiology: the cause of a disease.

Exacerbation: increase in the symptoms or severity of a disease Healing: the restoration to a normal mental or physical condition.

Health history: a written record of past and current health events, including illnesses, accidents and surgeries.

Holistic: the perspective that, in nature, organisms (including people) function as complete units that cannot be reduced to the sum of their parts; in people, all facets of their well-being are considered, including the mental, emotional, physical, spiritual, economic, environmental, social and energetic.

Homeostasis: state of dynamic equilibrium or balance in the body/mind; innately maintained by the processes of feedback and regulation.

Idiopathic: conditions without a clear or apparent cause.

Illness: the state of being sick; an ailment.

Indication: any persuasive reason to do a specific therapeutic action Injury: trauma or damage to the body.

Injury: a trauma or damage to the body.

Local: relating only to a specific area of the body.

L: left

Massage therapy: the systematic therapeutic manipulation of the body's soft tissues by a specially trained therapist.

Naturopathic: a therapeutic system that does not use drugs but employs natural forces such as light, heat, air, water, nutrition and massage.

Nursing: the diagnosis and treatment of human responses to actual or potential health problems.

Objective: information that can be sensed or measured by an observer, for instance, a wart, bruise or range of motion; signs.

Observation: looking and listening carefully with attention to detail.

Oriental Medicine: a holistic therapeutic paradigm associated with the healing practices that originated in Asia, having central principles of Qi, or the life force, and the duality of Yin/Yang.

Orthopedic: the movement (or "locomotor") system of the body.

Palpation: the process of examining the body by applying one's hands to the body surface.

Paradigm: a philosophical and theoretical framework within which theories, laws and generalizations (and the experiments performed in support of them) are formulated.

Pathology: the study of the nature of diseases and the structural and functional changes produced by them; a deviation from health.

Petrissage: a kneading stroke in massage therapy.

Placebo: an inert substance that appears to be the same as the experimental substance but it actually has no known effects

Practice: in health care, the use of knowledge and skill to provide a service in the prevention, diagnosis and treatment of illness and the maintenance of health.

Primary care provider (PCP): a health professional who provides periodic check-ups, evaluates and diagnoses illnesses and coordinates the plan of treatment.

Professional liability: means the obligation of the professional to pay for damages resulting from the professional's acts of omission or commission involved in their contact with clients.

Prognosis: the prediction of the course and end of a disease, and the estimate of chance for recovery.

Pseudoscientific: using a set of ideas based on theories put forth as scientific when they are *not* scientific.

R: right

Referral: to send or direct for treatment, aid, information or decision.

Remission: a lessening of severity or abatement of symptoms.

Risk factors: conditions that make a negative event more likely, but they are not necessarily the cause.

ROM: range of motion.

Science: the intellectual process for using all of the mental and physical resources available in order to better understand, explain, quantify and predict normal and unusual phenomena

Scientific: using observation, measurement, accumulated data, and logical analysis of the findings to understand, predict and explain phenomena.

Sign: any objective evidence of illness or disordered function; signs are more or less definitive and obvious, and apart from the patient's impression, in contrast to symptoms which are more subjective.

Subacute: between acute and chronic, but with some acute features.

Subjective: information that is known directly only by the person who experiences it, for instance, fear, pain, anxiety, joy, etc.; symptoms.

Symptom: any subjective evidence of illness or disordered function.

Syndrome: a group of signs and symptoms of disordered function related to each other by means of some anatomic, physiologic or biochemical peculiarity; does not include a precise cause but provides a framework for investigation.

Systemic: relating to the entire body/mind.

Theory: a speculation, supposition, or assumption based on certain evidence or observations but lacking scientific proof; Synonym: hypothesis.

Therapeutic action: skillful behaviors, applied to help a person, which have medicinal, supportive or healing properties.

Therapeutic outcome: the effect your work has on the client. Therapy: treatment of a disease or pathological condition.

Traditional healing: any therapeutic system of social and/or biological methods, beliefs and values that are used by people of a particular family or culture and are passed from generation to generation.

Transference: the projection by a client of feelings, needs, or issues onto a therapist, instead of recognizing them as his or her own.

Treatment: any specific procedure used for the cure or amelioration of a disease or pathological condition.

Wkly: weekly

x: a common symbol meaning "times"

(Tabor's, 1998) used in this chapter refers to Tabor's Medical dictionary (http://www.tabers.com/tabersonline/ub/)

* * *

Chapter III

History and Theory of Reflexology

> Reflexology has a fascinating history from the tombs of Ancient Egypt to Cleopatra to the rediscovery of this lost art in the 1900's.

The History of Reflexology

Foot work practices have existed throughout the history of humankind. Remnants of foot work practices span time and place from the Physician's Tomb in Egypt of 2300 B.C. A high-ranking official during the time of the Egyptian Sixth Dynasty, 2323 to 2150 BCE, was buried in the ancient burial ground at Saqqara. His tomb is especially interesting to the medical professions as pictographs display multiple scenes of people undergoing medical treatment. Ankhmahor's tomb also holds a pictograph demonstrating work on the hands and feet.

Another Egyptian pictograph was found in the temple of Amen at Karnak during Ramses II reign of 1279-13 BCE and depicts a "healer tending to the feet of foot soldiers at the battle of Qadesh." It is thought that this foot therapy spread from Egypt through the Roman Empire. The Roman Emperor Octavian, 62-14 CE, mentions the foot massages Mark Antony, 83-30 BCE, gave to the Egyptian Queen Cleopatra VII, C. 69-30.

The modern history of reflexology is rooted in research about the reflex in Europe and Russia 125 years ago. The idea that a stimulus applied to the body produces a response was utilized as a therapeutic tool by British physicians and researchers who applied heat, cold, plasters, and herbal poultices to one part of the body to influence another. While such uses did not take root in the medical communities in the United States and Great Britain, the furthering of such ideas for therapeutic use continued in Germany and Russia throughout this century.

Russian physicians of the early 1900's followed the reflex research of Nobel Prize winner Ivan Pavlov to create Reflex Therapy. Their basic idea, to influence reflexes and thus brain-organ dynamics, survives as a medical practice today.

To physician researchers, such as Vladimir Bekterev who coined the word "reflexology" in 1917, *an organ experiences illness because it receives the wrong instructions from the brain.* By interrupting the body's misguided instructions, the reflex therapist prompts the body to behave in a better manner. Conditioning of better behavior is achieved by the application of a series of such interruptions.

American physiotherapist Eunice Ingham kept alive a specific practice, that of foot reflexology. She accomplished this by traveling around the country teaching groups of people, perpetuating a grassroots enthusiasm for the subject in the United States. A community of reflexology users emerged. Legal questions were raised about the practice of medicine without a license. Ms. Ingham's book of 1945 ascribed the workings of reflexology to the nervous system. The revised work published in 1954, deleted any such mention. the explanation of the workings of reflexology took on metaphorical terms that were to color the practice for decades to come.

The term reflexology itself was considered illegal until a legal skirmish over the publication of Mildred Carter's book *Helping Yourself with Foot Reflexology* in 1970. The U.S. postal Service asked that the publisher cease and desist publication of the book on the grounds that it consisted of the practice of medicine without a license.

The publisher's attorneys successfully defended the publication of the book. Subsequently the word could be used to describe one's practice; it was also used in the titles of books. The idea became widely disseminated as Mrs. Carter's book sold one million copies and became one of the best-selling titles ever for the publisher.

In the following quarter century, the idea gained informal sanctioning in the United States on a community level. Since then, practicing reflexologists have emerged, Some 30 reflexology books have been published, and the number of magazine articles published has climbed by 500 percent since 1982. Television appearances by reflexologists have increased by 500 percent since 1988.

The Theory Behind Reflexology

The underlying theory behind reflexology is that there are "reflex" areas on the feet and hands that correspond to specific organs, glands, and other parts of the body.

For example:
  * the tips of the toes reflect the brain.
  * the heart and chest are around the ball of the foot.
  * the liver, pancreas and kidney are in the arch of the foot.
  * low back and intestines are towards the heel.

Dr. William H. Fitzgerald, an ear, nose, and throat doctor, introduced this concept of "zone therapy" in 1915. American physiotherapist Eunice Ingram further developed this zone theory in the 1930's into what is now known as reflexology.

A scientific explanation is that the pressure may send signals that balance the nervous system or release chemicals such as endorphins that reduce pain and stress.

Reflexology is known to help with:
- Stress and stress-related conditions
- Tension headaches
- Digestive disorders
- Arthritis
- Insomnia
- Hormonal imbalances
- Sports injuries
- Menstrual disorders, such as premenstrual syndrome (PMS)
- Digestive problems, such as constipation
- Back pain

Reflexology is a popular alternative therapy. It promotes relaxation, improves circulation, reduces pain, soothes tired feet, and encourages overall healing.

Reflexology is also used for post-operative or palliative care. A study in the American Cancer Society journal found that one-third of cancer patients used reflexology as a complementary therapy.

Reflexology is recommended as a complementary therapy and should not replace medical treatment.

What is a typical reflexology treatment like?

A typical treatment is 45 minutes to 60 minutes long and begins with a consultation about your health and lifestyle.

You are then asked to remove your shoes and socks and sit comfortably in a reclining chair or on a massage table. Otherwise you remain fully clothed. The reflexologist will assess the feet and then stimulates various points to identify areas of tenderness or tension.

The reflexologist then uses brisk movements to warm the feet up. Then pressure is applied from the toes to the heel according to your comfort. Lotion or oil may be used throughout or not at all.

* * *

Chapter IV

Intuition For Therapists

As a reflexologist, it is your responsibility to ensure the comfort of your clients, making communication a vital part in an effective reflexology session. But what do you do when your client doesn't communicate? How will you know the appropriate techniques to perform when your client is offering you little or no feedback? Intuition, that's how.

Intuition doesn't rely on verbal communication; it's more of an internal knowledge. For reflexologists and other body workers, accessing your intuition is extremely important in order to be an effective healer. Balancing this spiritual insight with your physical knowledge of reflexology techniques will help guide you through a session by listening and responding to your client's body and sensing their needs, without saying a word. Many practitioner's that are drawn to energy work are already intuitive.

There are specific modalities (mainly energy work) that require the therapist to utilize their intuitive senses. The more skilled you become as a therapist, combined with a heightened awareness of your intuition, the easier it will be to let your hands guide you through a session without relying on the client for feedback. Think of intuition as your instinct. It comes naturally, and usually doesn't require much thought. It takes time and practice to become aware of this intuitive sense, so be patient and spend some time each day tapping into this spiritual sense.

As a bodywork professional, trusting yourself and your intuition is key; throw away any doubts you may have and simply learn to let this inner sense guide you. When your client is unable or unwilling to offer a response during a session, let everything else fall away and simply listen to the voice inside you.

What can you do when a client doesn't provide you with any verbal feedback?

How can you tailor treatments to meet their needs?

You can learn to develop your intuition so you can turn this difficult situation into a successful session.

Always remember that. . .

Every client is different.

Some clients will enter your healing space totally aware of their physical and emotional health barometer, while others only know that they feel good after a session. Communicating with your clients in order to cover such crucial aspects as comfortable pressure limits, body temperature, health history, description of physical sensations and the uncovering of emotions hidden in muscle tissue is integral to an effective session. Asking for and receiving feedback from your client enables the therapist to tailor their treatment to specific needs and wants. A challenge arises when the client does not offer feedback, or worse, is unaware of their current physical and/or emotional experience. This is when intuition can help guide a therapist through a successful session.

The ability to simultaneously combine input from our intuition and intellect is the premier mark of a gifted healer. Having the analytical skills and facts organized in the left brain can only get body workers so far, especially when approaching a client who is less than communicative. The ability to access the creative intuition from the right brain can guide the body worker in many areas, such as where pain originates, to choosing the best modality for any given client or in determining the right amount of time spent on a constricted muscle group.

The well-known style of Essalen massage incorporates intuition into its description, and gives a good understanding of the relationship between intuition and bodywork:

The practitioner brings a knowledge of strokes (many have roots in Swedish Massage), of muscles and bones, of movement, of listening to the body as well as the words. Prior to the session, he/she pays attention to his own physical comfort, and quiets down internal chatter to welcome inner guidance, or intuition. As he massages, the practitioner responds to the signs of relaxation: deepened breath, enhanced circulation, a sigh, perhaps flutters of the eyelids. Each session is unique, tailored by personal requests, comfort level, physical tension and release, the felt sense of intuition.

Many gentle and/or energetic modalities such as, Therapeutic Touch, Reiki and CranioSacral Therapy, require the practitioner to be still and aware in effort to connect with their intuitive sense.

Appreciating the subtle, yet definite force of each client's energetic needs, fosters a cross-over between the practitioner's right and left brains. This cross-over is the culmination of learned academics with sensed phenomena representing the most advanced form of healing.

Everyone experiences a continual stream of intuitive thoughts. Unfortunately, our culture has trained us to ignore such "right-brained" hype. As a result, many people ignore, discount or contradict their gut feelings. Developing intuition requires an initial awareness of its presence. Most people need time and practice to identify these thoughts when they surface to give them credence and volume instead of the well-practiced dismissal.

For reflexologists, a critical aspect in following their intuition is the ability to trust oneself. Another aspect of our cultural conditioning is to look to authorities or teachers for answers or directions. Learning to trust your intuition harbors the belief that listening to yourself will lead you well.

Doubt can arise for a practitioner mid-session. Examples include:

- What area or technique should I work next?
- Should I spend more time on this muscle group or that zone?
- Could this move be uncomfortable for my client?
- Can this client handle more pressure?

If the client is unable to provide the appropriate feedback to satisfy your doubt, ask for inner guidance.

Everyone possesses an intuitive voice that contains answers about healing. However, the volume of the intellect can be so loud as to drown out this inner voice. Devoting a few minutes each day to listening to your intuitive voice will help every therapist trust inner wisdom signals, propelling your skills from mediocre to expert.

Guidelines For Awakening Intuition *

INTENTION: The first requirement for consciously awakening intuition is a clear intention to do so. Intuition is already within you, but to awaken it you have to value it and INTEND to develop it.

TIME: Your willingness to devote time to tuning in to your intuition, making a space for its unfolding in your life, is part of valuing and developing it.

RELAXATION: Letting go of physical and emotional tension gives intuition the space to enter your conscious awareness.

SILENCE: Intuition flourishes in silence. Learning to quiet the mind is therefore part of the training for awakening intuition. Various meditative practices are useful in learning to maintain the necessary inner silence.

HONESTY: Willingness to face self-deception and to be honest with yourself and others is essential. Creating any kind of smokescreen interferes with clear vision. Giving up pretenses is a big step in awakening intuition.

RECEPTIVITY: Learning to be quiet and receptive allows intuition to unfold. Too much activity or conscious programming gets in the way of intuitive awareness that emerges when a receptive attitude is cultivated.

SENSITIVITY: Finely tuned sensitivity to both inner and outer processes provides more information and expands intuitive knowing. Sensitivity to energy awareness and the quality of experience is particularly useful.

NONVERBAL PLAY: Drawing, music, movement, clay, and other forms of nonverbal expression done in a spirit of play, rather than for the purpose of goal-oriented achievement, provide excellent channels for activating intuitive, right-hemisphere functions.

TRUST: Trusting the process, trusting yourself, trusting your experience, are the keys to trusting and developing your intuition.

OPENNESS: If you are afraid of being seen, you may close up and then be unable to see. Being open to all experiences, both inner and outer, gives intuition the space it needs to develop fully.

COURAGE: Fear gets in the way of direct experience and often generates deception. Your willingness to experience and confront your fears will facilitate the expansion of intuition.

ACCEPTANCE: A nonjudgmental attitude, an acceptance of things as they are, including self-acceptance, allows intuition to function freely.

LOVE: Opening your heart to feelings of nonjudgmental love and compassion allows you to see into the nature of things. Emotional empathy and intuitive identification are facilitated by love and compassion.

NONATTACHMENT: The willingness to let things be as they are, rather than trying to make them be the way you would like them to be, or the way you think they should be, allows intuition to emerge. You can see things as they are only when desires and fears are out of the way.

DAILY PRACTICE: Intuitive awareness grows with daily attention.

If you discount or neglect it most of the time and only want it to perform occasionally, it may not respond.

JOURNAL KEEPING: Keeping a record of intuitive flashes, hunches, insights, and images that come to mind spontaneously at any time of the day or night, can help stabilize and validate them.

SUPPORT GROUP: Finding one, two, or more friends with whom you can share your interest in the development of intuition, as well as your successes, failures, hopes, and fears, can facilitate and accelerate the process of development. Sharing experience with someone who is willing to listen without judging or interpreting is very useful.

ENJOYMENT: Following intuition does not always feel good. At times it may seem difficult and entail arduous work. At other times it may be effortless. Enjoying the creative resources of intuition is based on the intrinsic satisfaction of expanding consciousness, taking responsibility for your life, and surrendering to your own true nature.

* Source: Awakening Intuition by Frances Vaughan, Anchor Books, 1979, New York, New York

* * *

Notes:

Chapter V

Ear Reflexology

The term *Reflexology* is commonly thought to only apply to the feet; however Auricular Therapy, or Ear Reflexology, has been around since prior to the Julian calendar. It has only recently been rediscovered and is an important tool for many professional Reflexologists.

A History of Auricular Therapy

The classic Traditional Chinese Medicine (TCM) text, *Huang Di Nei Jing*, also known as the Yellow Emperor's Medicine Classic, describes a correlation between the auricle and the body. Dating one hundred years before the Julian calendar, this is the oldest known reference to the ear reflecting other body parts for a therapeutic purpose.

There is mention of pains being treated long before the coming of the modern age through the use of Zone Therapy.

In Hippocrates' time, around 400 BC, descriptions of back pain being relieved through tiny burns to certain zones in the ears may show that the auricular theory traveled extensively.

By the time of the Tang Dynasty, 618-907 AD, there were twenty therapeutic points in the ears available to auricular acupuncture. Turning up in 1637 AD, a Portuguese physician, Zaratus Lusitanus, published a case study of his treatment for a patient with painful back problems using small burns on the ears.

In the 1950s Dr. Paul Nogier, a French physician, had patients turning up with burn marks on their ears. They were receiving treatment from a folk healer for back pain. Nogier studied the patterns and worked out the *reflex cartography* of the ears and presented his findings at a symposium in 1956, calling it *Auricle Therapy*.

Modern Auricular Therapy is utilized by Asian bodywork modalities such as Shiatsu and Anma, as well as by Acupuncturists, and of course Reflexologists. Bill Flocco, founder of the American Academy of Reflexology, has popularized Ear Reflexology through his method of Reflexology: Foot, Hand, Ear Reflexology.

This style of Reflexology incorporates all three reflex maps into a single session – the practitioner uses only finger and thumb techniques and may spend more time on one pair of maps than the other two.

The Application of Ear Reflexology

Ear Reflexology is administered through thumb and finger pressure techniques applied to the external ears. When used alongside other reflex maps an Ear Reflexology treatment may last 10-15 minutes. As a stand alone treatment a Reflexologist may offer a 30 minute Ear Reflexology session.

Contraindications

Contraindications for Ear Reflexology include psoriasis or eczema sores that are open or other wounds to the ears that are not yet healed. A session should be postponed until the issue clears up or an alternative map, such as the hands, may be used. Clients with hearing assistance devices may choose to remove an external hearing aid for a session. Those with internal, or implanted, devices will best know if external stimulus to the ear will be appropriate for them.

Simple Ear Reflexology Routine

A quick routine for the ears as a self-help method can be done while seated.

The fore fingers and thumbs can wrap around each ear lobe and gently "milk" downwards towards the shoulders. This rubbing can be drawn all the way to the apex of the ear – upwards to the ceiling and crown of the head. In this quick routine the reflexes for the neck, shoulders and spine are covered.

Anatomy of the Ear

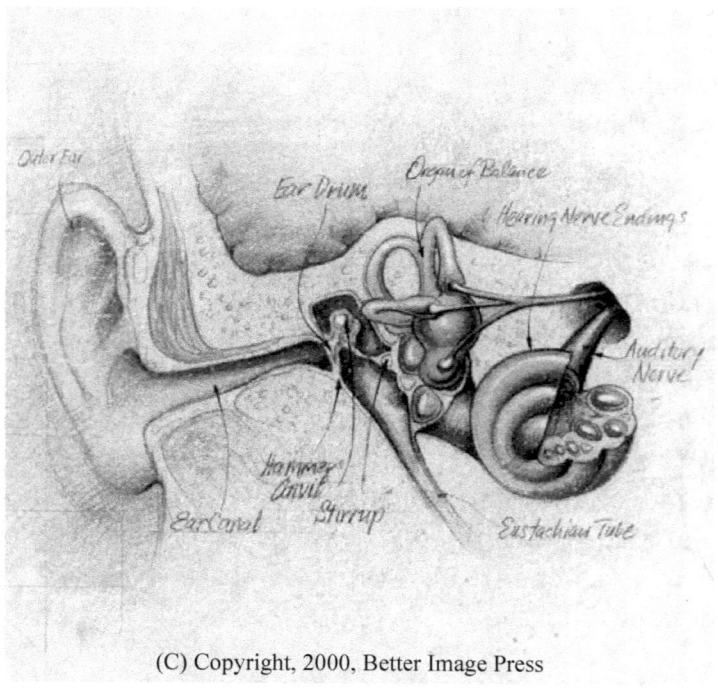

* * *

Notes:

Chapter VI

Anatomy (of the feet)

The human foot is one of the best-engineered parts of the body. Each foot has 33 joints, 8 arches, 26 bones, 100+ muscles, ligaments, and tendons that all work together to distribute body weight and allow movement. Unfortunately, many people pay no attention to their feet – until they start to hurt.

Foot disorders must be diagnosed and treated early, before they become very painful and incapacitating. In some cases, some painful foot abnormalities are already warning signs of even more serious ailments such as diabetes, circulatory disorders, and nerve problems.

Bones of the leg

A. Tibia, Latin meaning *reed pipe*
   1. tibial plateau
   2. medial tibial condyle
   3. lateral tibial condyle
   4. intercondylar eminence
   5. tibial tuberosity
   6. medial surface
   7. fibular notch
   8. medial malleolus

B. Fibula, from Latin meaning *pin* or *clasp*
   1. head
   2. lateral malleolus

Bones of the Foot and Ankle

A. Tarsals
   1. The term *tarsal* means "pile of rocks" which is what this group of seven bones look like.
   2. The tarsals of the ankle are analogous to the carpals of the wrist.
   3. The tarsals are irregularly shaped bones.

The joints between them are called intertarsal joints, they are gliding joints.

Not a lot of movement occurs between any two tarsals but the combined movement of the intertarsal joints plus the movement at the talocrural joint result in the four movements of the ankle.

4. **Joints that make up the ankle**

   a. Talocrural: hinge joint formed by the articulation of the inferior aspects of the tibia and fibula with the superior aspect of the talus.

   b. Intertarsal joints: gliding joints formed by the articulation of each tarsal with its neighboring tarsals.

5. **Movements of the ankle**

   a. *plantar flexion:* pointing the toes down.

   b. *dorsiflexion:* bringing the dorsal part of the foot up toward the anterior leg.

   c. *inversion:* bringing the medial longitudinal arch up and the lateral aspect of the foot down so that the souls of the feet face each other.

   d. *eversion:* bringing the medial longitudinal arch down and the lateral aspect of the foot

6. **Name and location of the seven tarsal bones**

    a. Talus: most superior of the tarsals, located directly inferior to the distal aspects of the tibia and fibula.

    b. Calcaneus: largest and most posterior of the tarsals, makes up the heel.

    c. Navicular: distal to the taius at the high point of the medial longitudinal arch. The three cuneiforms are distal to the navicular

    d. Cuboid: distal to the calcaneus at the lateral aspect of the transverse arch

    e. Cuneiforms: three bones distal to the navicular, they are distinguished from each other both as cuneiform 1, 2 and 3 (from medial to lateral) or as the medial, intermediate and lateral cuneiform.

B. Metatarsals

    1. Like in the hand, the long bones of the foot that are distal to the tarsals are named the metatarsals. From medial to lateral they are metatarsal 1,2,3,4 and 5.

    2. Each has a head at the distal end and a base at the proximal end.

The heads of the metatarsals make up what is commonly referred to as the ball of the foot. The heads are where the majority of one's weight is when standing "on the toes."

C. Phalanges (singular phalanx)

1. Like in the hand, digit 1 of the foot (called the big toe, the great toe or the hallucis) is made up of two phalanges, a proximal and a distal.

2. Digits 2-5 each have three phalanges, a proximal, an intermediate and a distal.

3. Like the metatarsals, the phalanges also have a head at the distal end and a base at the proximal end.

D. Joints of the foot

1. Tarsometatarsal joints: formed by the articulation of the distal aspect of the distal tarsals and the base of the metatarsals. Very little movement occurs at these joints.

2. Metatarsophalangeal joints: formed by the heads of the metatarsals and the bases of the proximal phalanges. These joints can do flexion, extension, adduction and abduction.

3. Interphalangeal joints

    a. digit 1 has one interphalangeal joint between its two phalanges.

    b. digits 2-5 have a proximal interphalangeal joint between the proximal and the intermediate phalanges.

    c. digits 2-5 also have a distal interphalangeal joint located between the intermediate and distal phalanges.

    d. the actions of the interphalangeal joints are flexion and extension

E. Arches

1. The arch is the strongest structure in nature. It is logical to find three of these structures on the foot since the foot, with its relatively small surface area, must support and balance the entire weight of the body.

2. The largest arch is the medial longitudinal arch. It runs lengthwise on the foot from just posterior to the middle of the calcaneus through the navicular and the three cuneiforms to the head of metatarsals 1, 2 and 3.

3. Running parallel to the medial longitudinal arch is the **lateral longitudinal** arch. It goes from just anterior to the middle of calcaneus through the Cuboid to the heads of metatarsals 4 and 5.

4. The **transverse arch** runs perpendicular to the two longitudinal arches and includes the three cuneiforms and the Cuboid.

5. **functions** of the **arches**

   a. transmit the weight of the body to the ground

   b. absorb shock

   c. aid in balance

   d. medial longitudinal arch transmits the weight of the body forward to the big toe when walking and running. In this action, it becomes a spring that helps to propel the body forward.

Anterior and Posterior Leg Bones

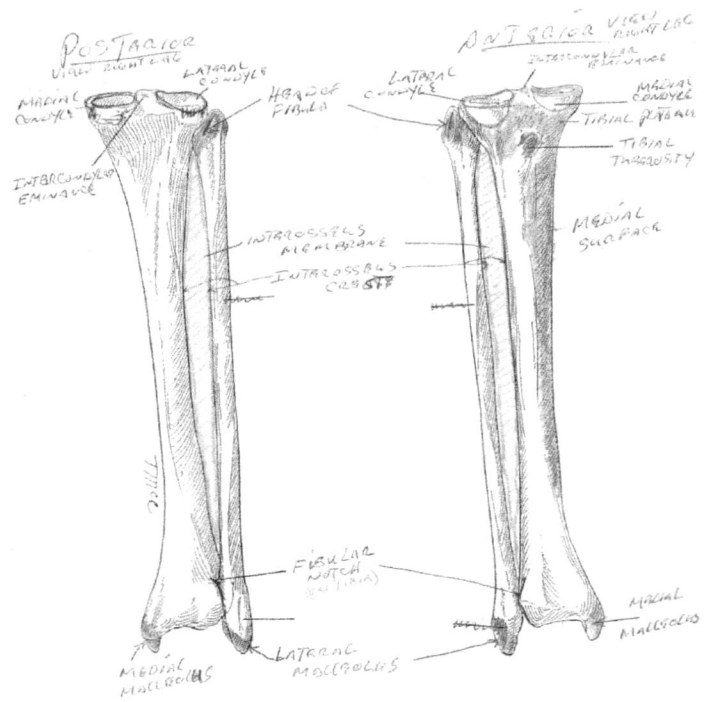

12.3 Posterior Leg   Fig. 12.4 Anterior Leg

Bones of the Foot

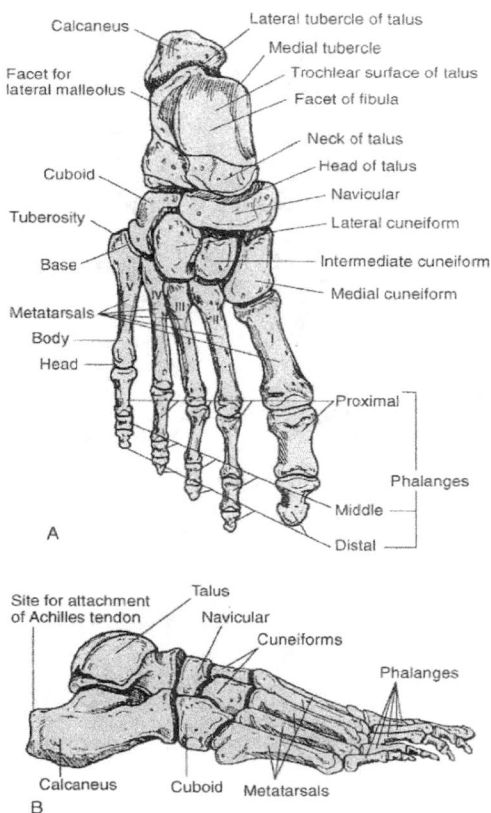

ABC's of Reflexology

Plantar Surface of the Foot

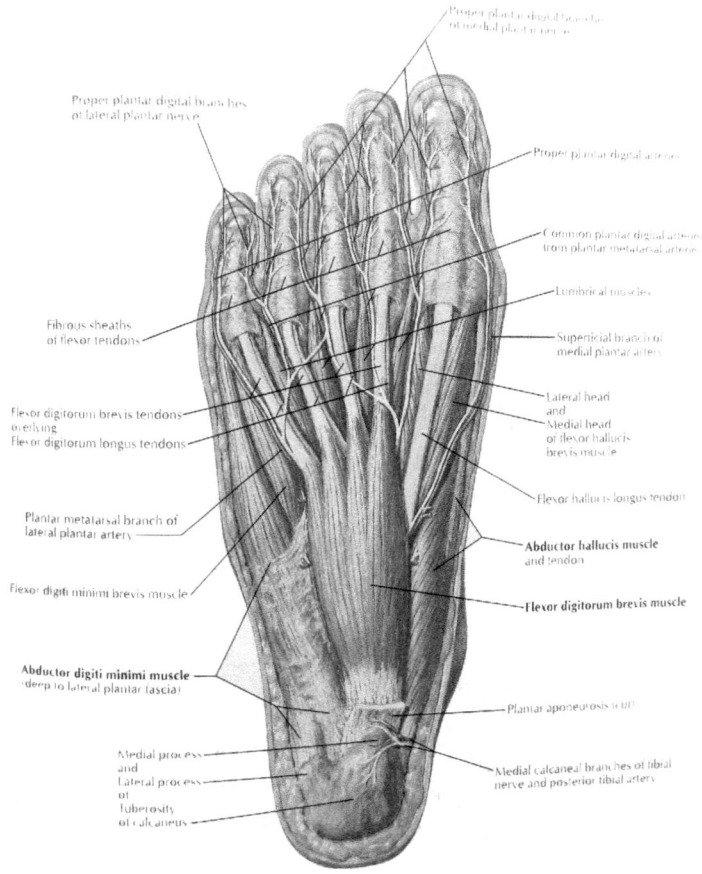

Proper plantar digital branches
of medial plantar nerve

Proper plantar digital branches
of lateral plantar nerve

Proper plantar digital arteries

Common plantar digital arteries
from plantar metatarsal arteries

Lumbrical muscles

Fibrous sheaths
of flexor tendons

Superficial branch of
medial plantar artery

Flexor digitorum brevis tendons
overlying
Flexor digitorum longus tendons

Lateral head
and
Medial head
of flexor hallucis
brevis muscle

Flexor hallucis longus tendon

Plantar metatarsal branch of
lateral plantar artery

Abductor hallucis muscle
and tendon

Flexor digiti minimi brevis muscle

Flexor digitorum brevis muscle

Abductor digiti minimi muscle
(deep to lateral plantar fascia)

Plantar aponeurosis (cut)

Medial process
and
Lateral process
of
Tuberosity
of calcaneus

Medial calcaneal branches of tibial
nerve and posterior tibial artery

(C) Copyright 2000, Better Image Press

66

Plantar Surface Showing Inflamation

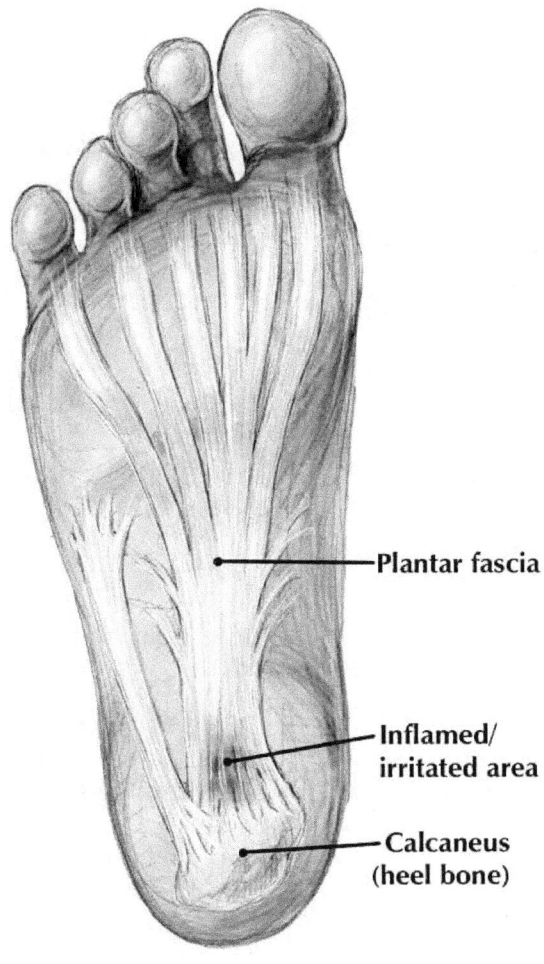

Plantar fascia

Inflamed/
irritated area

Calcaneus
(heel bone)

Plantar Surface Showing Flexors - 1

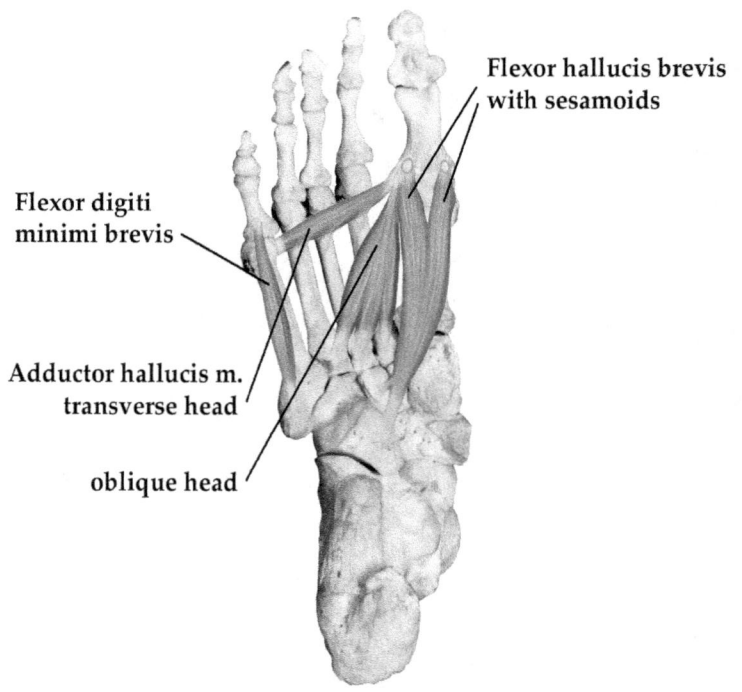

Flexor hallucis brevis
with sesamoids

Flexor digiti
minimi brevis

Adductor hallucis m.
transverse head

oblique head

Plantar Surface Showing Flexors - 2

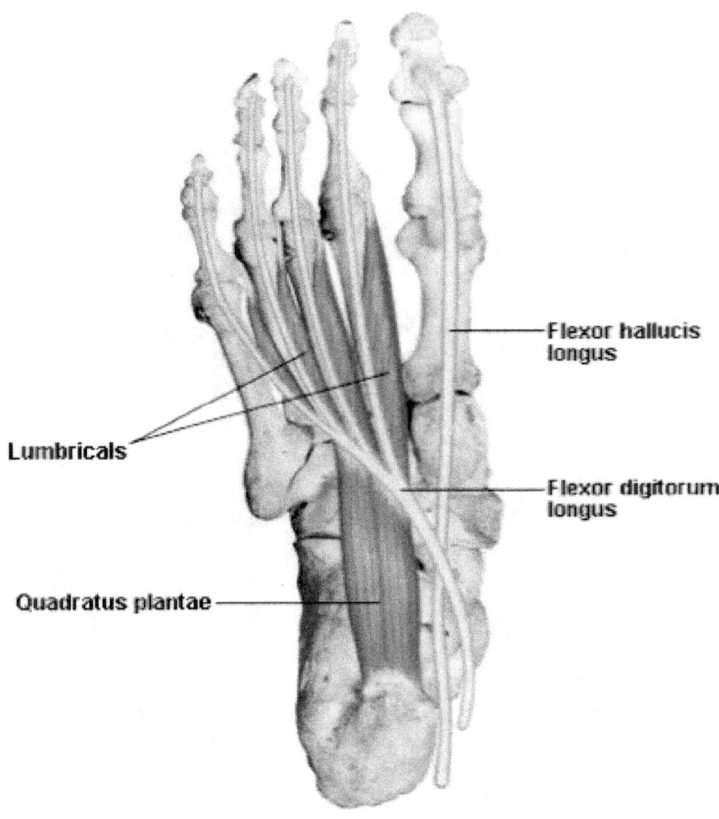

Flexor hallucis longus

Lumbricals

Flexor digitorum longus

Quadratus plantae

Muscles of the Foot and Leg

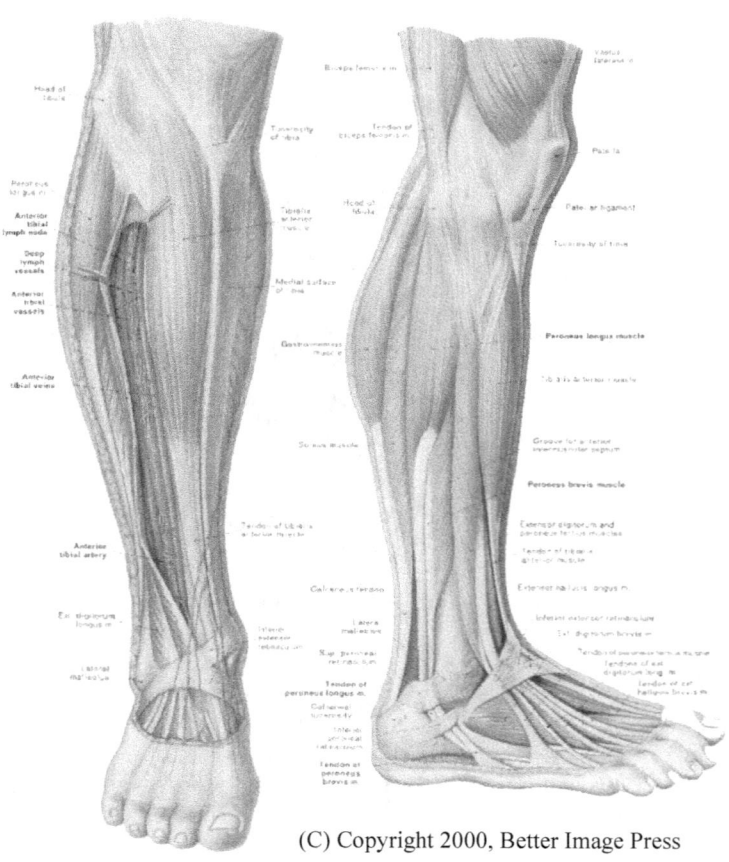

(Alternate View) Foot and Leg Muscles

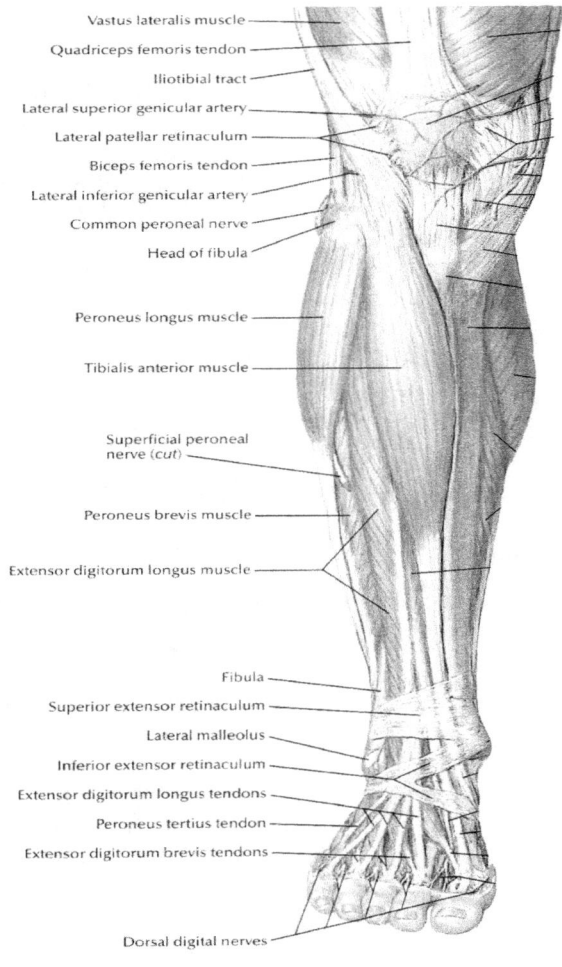

Vastus lateralis muscle

Quadriceps femoris tendon

Iliotibial tract

Lateral superior genicular artery

Lateral patellar retinaculum

Biceps femoris tendon

Lateral inferior genicular artery

Common peroneal nerve

Head of fibula

Peroneus longus muscle

Tibialis anterior muscle

Superficial peroneal nerve (cut)

Peroneus brevis muscle

Extensor digitorum longus muscle

Fibula

Superior extensor retinaculum

Lateral malleolus

Inferior extensor retinaculum

Extensor digitorum longus tendons

Peroneus tertius tendon

Extensor digitorum brevis tendons

Dorsal digital nerves

Notes:

Chapter VII

Anatomy of the Wrist and Hand

The wrist is formed primarily by the radius articulating with the Scaphoid and Lunate, and less so the Triquetrum.

The intercarpal joints are the joints between the carpal bones. A small amount of movement can occur at these joints.

Actions

a. flexion/extension
b. abduction/adduction (radial deviation/ulnar deviation) carpometacarpal joints, formed by the articulations between the carpals and the base of the metacarpals.

a. most of the carpometacarpal joints have an insignificant amount of movement that occurs at them
b. the carpometacarpal joint of the thumb is the "saddle joint" of the thumb.

Six actions occur at this joint.
  i.   flexion/extension
  ii. abduction/ adduction
  iii. opposition
  iv. circumduction

metacarpophalangeal joints, formed by the articulations between the head of the metacarpals and the base of the proximal phalanges. Four actions occur at these joints.
a. flexion/extension
b. abduction/adduction

Interphalangeal Joints
a. digit I has one interphalangeal joint
b. proximal interphalangeal joints (PIP)
  i. formed by the articulation of the head of the proximal phalanx and the base of the middle phalanx
  ii. found on digits II-V
c. distal interphalangeal joints (DIP)
  i. formed by the articulation of the head of the middle phalanx and the base of the distal

ii. found on digits II-V
d. actions: flexion/extension

Carpals, from Latin meaning *wrist*

A. There are 8 small bones in each wrist called carpals. They are arranged in two rows of four bones each.

B. The carpals as a group form a curved shape like a flattened letter "U". The tendons of the extrinsic hand muscles pass through the hollow part of the curve, as does the median nerve. This curve formation is called the carpal tunnel. The structures running through the carpal tunnel are held in place by the transverse carpal ligament that is also called the flexor retinaculum.

C. Proximal row (lateral to medial)
    Scaphoid, articulates with the radius
    Lunate, articulates with the radius
    Triquetrum
    Pisiform

D. Distal row (lateral to medial)
    Trapezium: articulates with metacarpal I
    the transverse carpal ligament attaches to the tubercle of the trapezium
    Trapazoid, articulates with metacarpal II
    Capitate, articulates with metacarpal III
    Hamate, articulates with metacarpals IV and V.

The transverse carpal ligament attaches to the hook of the hamate.

II. **Metacarpals,** meta- means *beyond*

A. There are five metacarpals distinguished from each other with numerals I-V. The thumb side is I and the little finger side is V.
Landmarks, present on all five metacarpals
- base, at the proximal end
- shaft
- head, at the distal end

III. **Phalanges,** from the Greek meaning *soldiers in line for battle.*
(singular phalanx)

A. Digit I, the pollicis, or the thumb has two phalanges, a proximal phalanx and a distal phalanx.

B. Digits II - V have three phalanges, a proximal, middle and distal phalanx.

C. Landmarks
- base, proximal
- shaft
- head, distal

Muscles of the Arm and Shouldar

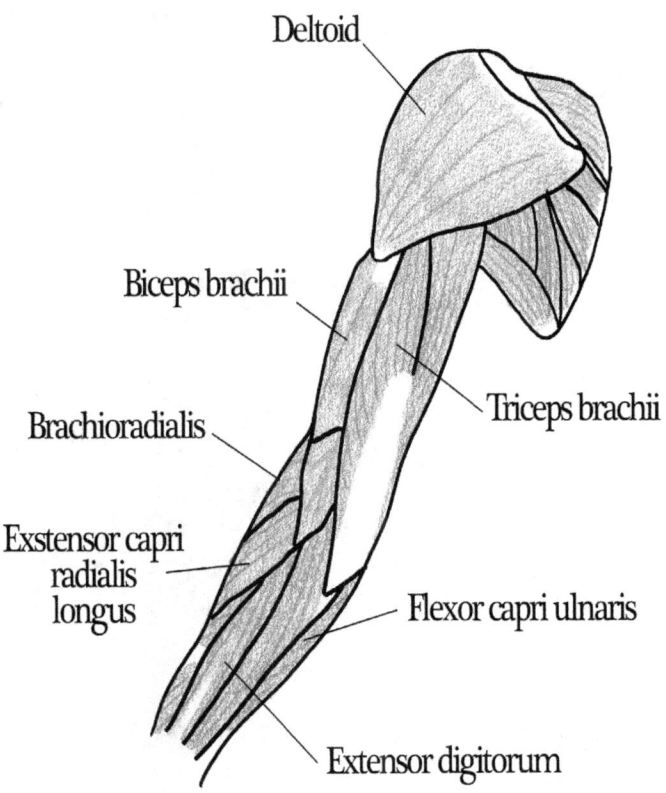

Deltoid

Biceps brachii

Brachioradialis

Exstensor capri
radialis
longus

Triceps brachii

Flexor capri ulnaris

Extensor digitorum

Muscles of the Arm

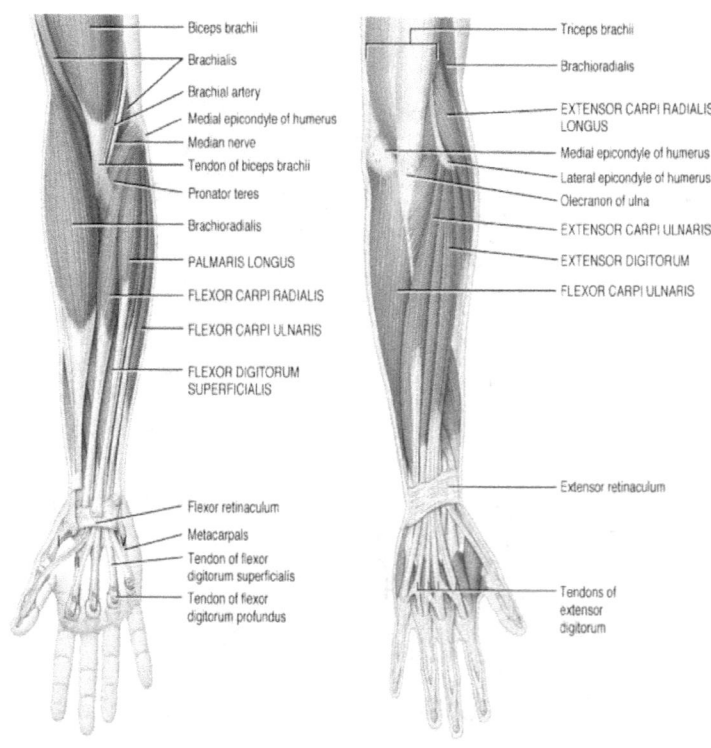

Anterior View   Posterior View

Bones of the Arm

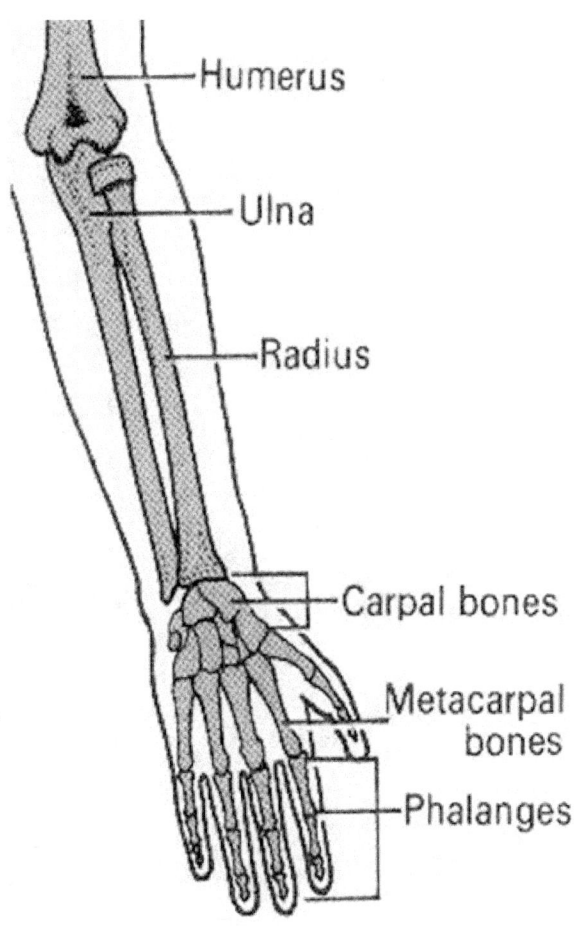

Anatomy of the Hand

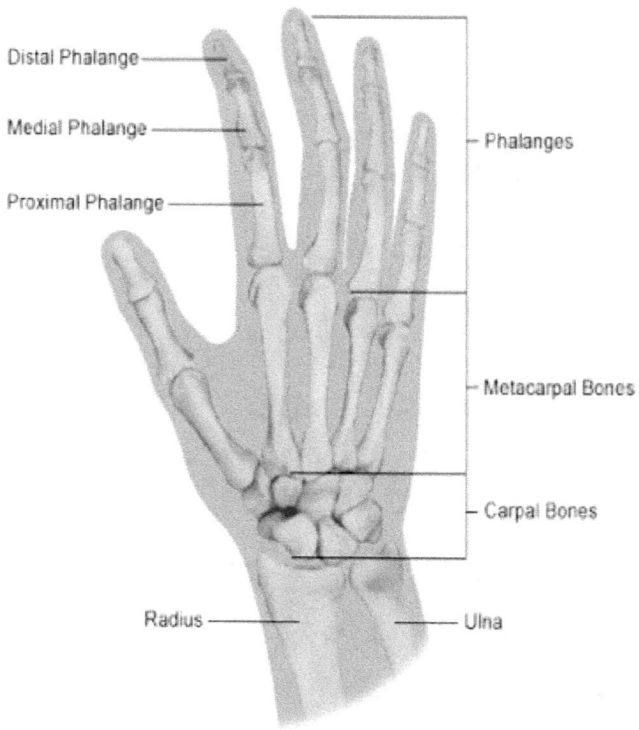

Distal Phalange

Medial Phalange

Proximal Phalange

Phalanges

Metacarpal Bones

Carpal Bones

Radius

Ulna

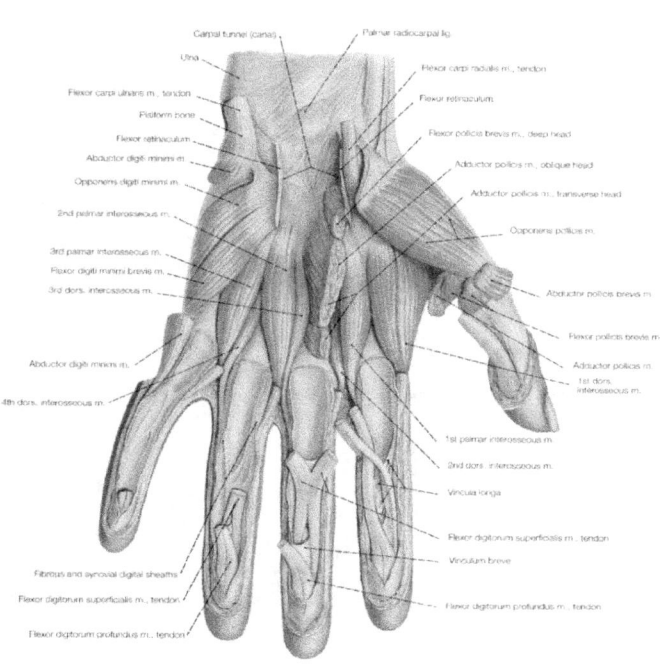

Carpal tunnel (canal)
Palmar radiocarpal lig.
Ulna
Flexor carpi radialis m., tendon
Flexor carpi ulnaris m., tendon
Flexor retinaculum
Pisiform zone
Flexor pollicis brevis m., deep head
Flexor retinaculum
Adductor pollicis m., oblique head
Abductor digiti minimi m.
Adductor pollicis m., transverse head
Opponens digiti minimi m.
Opponens pollicis m.
2nd palmar interosseous m.
3rd palmar interosseous m.
Flexor digiti minimi brevis m.
Abductor pollicis brevis m.
3rd dors. interosseous m.
Flexor pollicis brevis m.
Abductor digiti minimi m.
Adductor pollicis m.
1st dors. interosseous m.
4th dors. interosseous m.
1st palmar interosseous m.
2nd dors. interosseous m.
Vincula longa
Flexor digitorum superficialis m., tendon
Vinculum breve
Fibrous and synovial digital sheaths
Flexor digitorum superficialis m., tendon
Flexor digitorum profundus m., tendon
Flexor digitorum profundus m., tendon

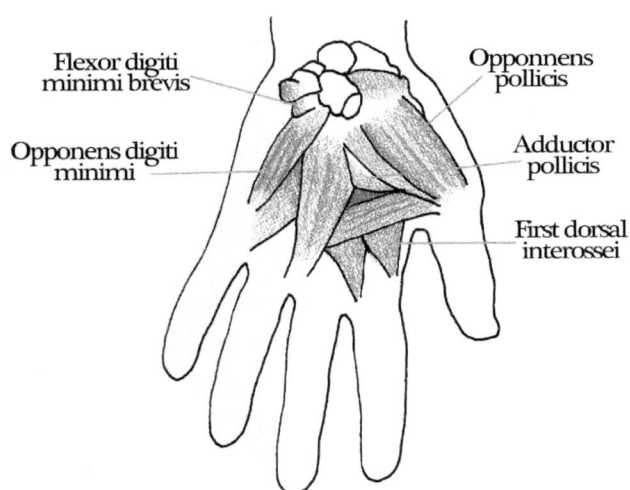

Flexor digiti minimi brevis

Opponnens pollicis

Opponens digiti minimi

Adductor pollicis

First dorsal interossei

Notes:

Chapter VIII

Mapping the Foot

REFLEXOLOGY FOOT CHART

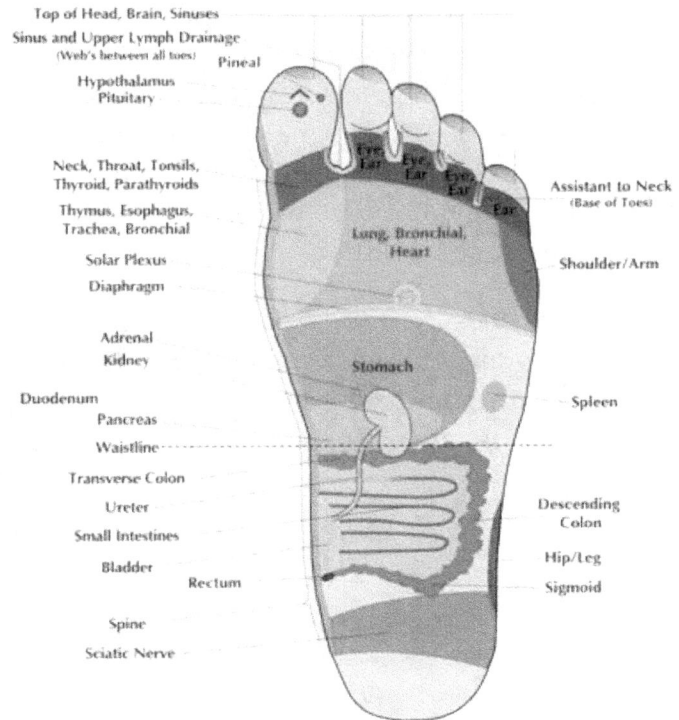

Top of Head, Brain, Sinuses
Sinus and Upper Lymph Drainage
(Web's between all toes)
Pineal
Hypothalamus
Pituitary

Neck, Throat, Tonsils,
Thyroid, Parathyroids
Thymus, Esophagus,
Trachea, Bronchial
Solar Plexus
Diaphragm

Adrenal
Kidney

Duodenum
Pancreas
Waistline
Transverse Colon
Ureter
Small Intestines
Bladder
Rectum
Spine
Sciatic Nerve

Eye, Ear
Eye, Ear
Eye, Ear
Ear

Lung, Bronchial,
Heart

Stomach

Assistant to Neck
(Base of Toes)

Shoulder/Arm

Spleen

Descending
Colon

Hip/Leg

Sigmoid

Mildred Carter's Foot Reflex Chart

So who is Mildred Carter and why do we use her foot chart? A very good question that we will answer here.

Mildred Carter was not a doctor, not an MD, DO or Ph.D. but spent forty years helping others through the use of reflexology. It is said that she cured aches and pains, not only in the feet but throughout the body through the application of reflexology. The lady had a remarkable record of providing relief and healing. During her forty years of practicing reflexology, she also wrote several books. Her titles, six or more, are available on Amazon. When asked why she used reflexology, she answered "Because the feet and hands contain reflexes which lead like telephone lines to all parts of the body, and by pressing them, you help restore normal circulation and health to congested areas"

Other persons besides Mildred, have mapped the foot, you can follow one of the other accepted ways or discover your own mapping system that works best for you. There is no one way that works best for everyone.

Inside View

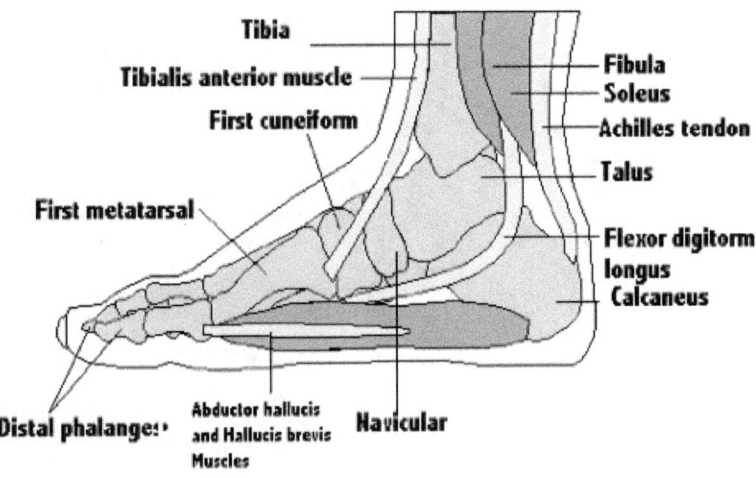

Tibia

Tibialis anterior muscle

First cuneiform

First metatarsal

Fibula
Soleus
Achilles tendon

Talus

Flexor digitorm longus
Calcaneus

Distal phalanges

Abductor hallucis and Hallucis brevis Muscles

Havicular

Outside View

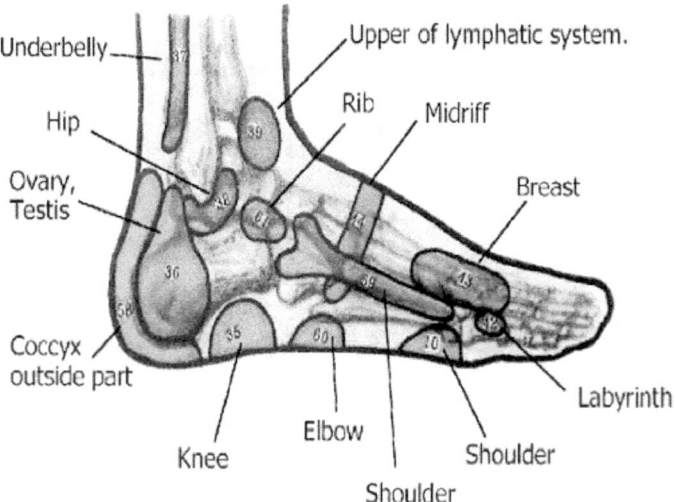

Underbelly

Upper of lymphatic system.

Hip

Rib

Midriff

Ovary,
Testis

Breast

Coccyx
outside part

Labyrinth

Knee

Elbow

Shoulder

Shoulder

The Acupuncture Meridians in the Foot

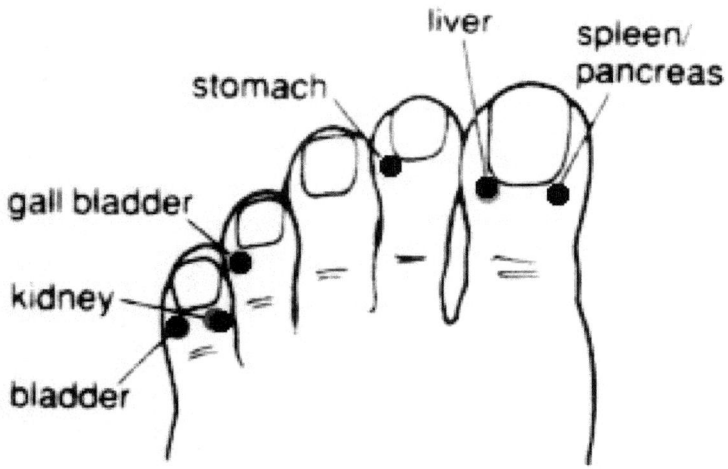

There are six meridians represented in the feet, specifically the toes. Using a basic knowledge of the meridians during reflexology, a reflexologist can have a better understanding of a client's condition. The meridians of feet are the spleen/pancreas, the liver, the stomach, the gallbladder, the kidney, and the bladder.

Meridians and reflexes often cross paths. Reflexology includes the stimulation of points along meridian lines. Zones connect with meridians throughout a reflexology session, giving further explanation to problem areas that have manifested on the feet.

The liver meridian begins in the leg and works in conjunction with the gallbladder and lung meridians. The liver meridian receives energy from the gallbladder line and transmits it to the lung pathway. This line starts between the first and second toe, runs along the inside of the leg, past the groin and bladder, touches the ribs, and ends in the chest. Changes in this meridian may be indicated by jaundice, fatigue, swelling of the liver, intestinal disorders, allergies, and headaches. This is a yin pathway associated with the element wood.

Zone Therapy

> **Zone Therapy is the Origin of hand and foot reflexology.**

This ancient therapy can be traced to the Egyptians. It is the origin of hand and foot reflexology. The zones also have a relationship to the acupressure circuitry. Zone therapy is a simple therapy. Anyone can do it.

With zone therapy, the body is divided by vertical lines into five zones on the left side and five zones on the right side. These zones relate to all parts of the body within each zone. The fingers and toes affect corresponding parts of the body and are the primary areas of treatment. Zone therapy works more directly on nerve endings that are connected with organs along the zones. This therapy is a very effective technique for pain release.

Primary emphasis is on the hands and feet, with a focus being on the fingers and toes. These parts of the body have the least depth to them. Nerve endings in these areas are near the surface and thus more accessible. The procedure is to press down using a circular, rolling motion. Look for the tender spots, using a constant kind of pressure. Begin with a light probe. If no tenderness is found, gently and slowly pressing deeper until the tenderness is found. Key on sensitivity. Apply pressure on the upper and lower surfaces as well as the sides of the fingers and toes. Do one area at a time, massaging all tender spots. When starting, pinpoint massage an area only for a few seconds, then let the area rest while you massage another spot. Keep coming back for a few seconds each time until the sensitivity is gone.

Do not over-massage at the beginning; proceed slowly.

Pinching the thumb and index finger together are the best instruments for fine in-depth stimulation. Pressure may also be applied with a blunt point applicator like a pencil with a rubber eraser. Clothespins may be used to apply strong, steady pressure. Pocket combs can be used along a wide area, clenching the fist to press the teeth of the comb against the inner surfaces of the fingers.

When working, cover all possible zones for a specific organ. Strong pressure on the tip of the thumb or big toe affects the whole first zone. Similar pressure on the tips of the other fingers and toes will affect corresponding zones. For example, an organ like the liver lies in all five zones on the right side and the eyes correspond with the three middle fingers and toes. The eyes relate to zones 3, 4, and 5. Pain anywhere in a particular zone will be lessened through pressure on the corresponding finger and toe. Pressure applied on the outside of the fingers and toes will be felt on the front of the body. Pressure on the inside of the fingers and the bottom of the toes will be expressed in the back.

Stimulate each tender spot at first for a maximum of 30 seconds. Increase pressure when tolerance has been established. Be persistent. For maximum effect, apply pressure for 30 seconds to four minutes, depending on the severity of the tenderness. Any tenderness is an indication of some degree of congestion in the associated zone. There is little written information on Zone Therapy. This is an opportunity to experiment, using your sensitivity and intuition.

Zone line – Organ Relationship

Center Zone Line 1	Thumbs & big toes	Pituitary, pineal, brain, hypothalamus, thyroid, sinuses, larynx, nose, trachea, tongue, esophagus, thymus, heart, spine, intestine, large intestine, pancreas, breast, small intestine, large intestine, prostate
Left Zone Line 2	Index finger & 2nd toe	Brain, eye, adenoids, lungs, heart, stomach, spleen, pancreas, breast, small intestine, large intestine
Left Zone Line 3	Middle finger & 3rd toe	Brain, eye, lung, breast, stomach, spleen, pancreas, kidney, adrenal gland, small intestine, large intestine
Left Zone Line 4	Ring Finger & 4th toe	Brain, eye, lung, breast, large intestine, ovaries
Left Zone Line 5	Little finger & 5th toe	Ears
Right Zone 2	Index finger & 2nd toe	Brain, eye, lung, breast, liver, small intestine, large intestine, adenoids
Right Zone 3	Middle finger & 3rd toe	Brain, eye, breast, liver, gall bladder, kidney, small intestine, large intestine, adrenal gland
Right Zone 4	Ring finger & 4th toe	Brain, eye, main lymphatic duct, breast, liver, lung, large intestine, ileo-cecal valve, appendix
Right Zone 5	Little finger & 5th toe	Ear

Notes:

Chapter IX

Basic Foot Techniques

The basic techniques to be covered in this chapter are the following.

a. Greeting the foot
b. Thumb & finger walking
c. Side to Side
d. Spinal twist
e. Lung press
f.   Ankle/toe Rotation

Begin with the right foot

a. **Greet the Foot**

Grasp the foot. Hold and press into the foot, Examine the foot, make sure there are no cuts or bruises. Also, check for knots and any crystal deposits. Using a baby wipe, it is advantageous to wipe each foot before beginning.

b. **Thumb and finger walking.**

Thumb walking is done on the fleshy side of the foot. Thumb walk all five zones. Finger walking is best for bony areas on the top of the foot and around the ankle.

c. **Side to side.**

Rock the foot from side to side by holding the heel in the palm of your hands, Rotate gently.

d. **Spinal twist.**

Hold the foot stationary at the arch. The webbing of your hand should be on should be on the inside edge of the foot. Place the second hand on the foot beside the first. Thumbs being next to each other. Gently twist back and forth. Keep your arms straight and elbows lock. Repeat several times then move both hands toward the toes until you have worked the entire foot.

e. **Lung press.**

Grasp the top of the foot just beneath the toes. Make a fist and press your knuckles into the foot This is done several times.

f. **Ankle rotation.**

Ankle rotations stretch and loosen the foot muscles and improve circulations to the ankles. By rotating the foot in a complete circle, you are providing both exercise and relaxation to the four major muscle groups that control the foot movements. Support the heel in one hand, thumb on the outside of the ankle, fingers on the inside. Grasp the top of the foot in your other and slowly and gently rotate the ankle several times in one direction and then in the other direction.

g. **Toe rotation.**

This technique will increase the flexibility of the toes and also loosen the muscles around the neck and shoulders. Support the foot gently with one hand, thumb on the sole of the foot, fingers wrapped around the top of the foot. Using your thumb and index finger close to the base of each joint, gently stretch each toe. Rotate each toe both clockwise and counter-clockwise, and repeat these steps.

Notes

Because of the importance of the large toe, I rotate it 15 times. The other toes usually are rotated at least 5 times.

Chapter X

Basic Hand Techniques

As with the Basic Foot Techniques, there are several Basic Hand Techniques. Sadly, there is just not enough space to cover all of them in this book and as with any practice, you will discover that there are certain techniques that you use over and over and some that you will never use. Personal preferences will always come into play. What we don't cover in this book will be, most likely, covered by others.

a. Finger pull
b. Side to Side
c. Rotation
d. Palm Rock
e. Hand Stretch
f. Palm Mover
g. Working The Fingers

a. **Finger pull**

Hold your client's wrist to support the hand. Gently and slowly stretch and squeeze each finger individually, working from the knuckle to the tip. Make circular pressures around each joint, using your thumb and forefinger. Gently flex and extend each finger and thumb joint with your thumb and forefinger. Circle around the thumb and fingers individually, both clockwise. Now circle them both counterclockwise.

b. **Side to side**

Place your hands on each side of the hand, palm facing you. Slot your thumbs in between   the thumb and little finger and rotate.

c. **Rotation**

In rotation, the tip of the thumb is placed directly on the point to be rotated. Using your hands to practice on, turn a palm up and find the space just below the little finger. Whatever palm you choose to work on, let it rest cupped in the other palm. The fingers of the holding hand, which is also the working hand, rest under the knuckles. The thumb is going to work on the palm surface from the little finger side. Feel under the little finger, on the palm surface. Find the undersurface of the knuckle bone and place your thumb on it. Back up to the edge of the hand and gently thumb walk over the bone, thumb walking in along the ball of the hand. You are walking horizontally across the palm.

This thumb-walking movement will take about three tiny inchworm bites to reach past this bone. Notice how the tip of the thumb drops into a space after the joint bone is passed over. If you have gone too far, you will find another bony bump, not quite as big as the first. First, hold the hand steady. Then gently circle in a small rotating motion on this area. Staying right here, continue this move for about the count of three. Now press and actually rotate the hand a little, moving it around as the thumb holds the spot. The moving of the hand is minimal. The movement of the hand is to allow the thumb to move in deeply without too much force. To transition from this, move forward in a thumb walk along the rest of the area being worked.

d. Thumb Walking

Thumb walking is the main movement made during a reflexology treatment. Apply steady, even pressure, moving along slowly over each area. The thumb is a tiny lever, touching the fine-point reflex areas in the most effective way. The nail must be short and neat with smooth edges so there is no dragging or digging on the foot.

Don't be concerned with identifying any of the reflex points. That will come later. You must learn how to walk before you can run. To practice this technique on your own - place one hand, palm down, flat on a table and let your other hand rest gently rest on top of it, palm down.

Let your thumb rest at the top of the hand by the first knuckle joint and your fingers loosely rest above this. (You may use either thumb to practice this move, as you will interchange thumbs and fingers during a session.) See how the top thumb touches with the tip and outside while resting on the top surface of the bottom hand. Bend this thumb up now so it is flexed at the first joint. This will allow the tip of the thumb to be on the skin with the remainder of the thumb bent up.

Push off with this thumb on the surface below so that the pad comes in contact with the skin. When doing this, your thumb will once again lie flat while the rest of the hand lies slightly across the surface with the fingers relaxed and wrapped easily around the outer edge of the hand. Pull the thumb back up into a bent position, hold down on this spot, and then move forward again.

The thumb continues to perform this creeping motion, You may notice that more of your thumb surface comes into play as you walk along (This is normal). The movement continues with small inching movements across the top of the hand. When you work across the top surface of the resting hand, the fingers (of the active hand) will be resting along the top of the resting hand above the knuckles. Each movement must be slow and controlled. Do not rush.

* * *

Chapter XI

Practice

Training, Certification and Licensing

As of 2014, the state of Arizona does not require reflexologists who focus solely on the hands and feet to obtain a massage license (This only apples if the client is fully clothed). If you intend to offer massage therapy, or if the client is unclothed, even if covered by a sheet), you will be required to obtain a massage license.

Obtaining first rate training and certification will not only help you establish your practice, but can give you a competitive advantage over your competition.

While undergoing training, consider volunteering at local nursing homes, gyms, hospitals and clinics as a way to get your name out there and gain experience.

Business License

Determine the scope and expansion possibilities for your reflexology practice. If you intend to operate from your home, either visiting your clients at their home or having them come to yours, you may operate as a sole proprietor (though you will need to contact your local zoning authority and homeowner's association to ensure that you can legally operate your practice from your home).

In that case, you will need to apply for a "Doing Business As" permit. The city of Tucson doesn't issue a generic business license. If you intend to open your own facility and hire employees, you will want to establish a limited liability company, which must be registered with the Secretary of State. You'll also want to purchase a liability insurance policy for your home or facility. Register with a professional organization such as the ABMP and get insured through them.

Location

Look to rent space in a reputable spa or clinic. Contact spa and clinic managers to pitch your practice and explain how having a reflexologist on board will boost business. When joining a team, ensure that the manager has all of the proper licenses, training and insurance and that he and his staff demonstrate the type of customer service that you subscribe to. Check, also, with Chiropracters and other doctors. If you intend to operate from home, set aside a room of the home for use as your home office and work area. Before you obtain a lease for rental space, calculate in detail, all of your enticipated regular business expenses and the rates you will charge in order to anticipate your expected gross income. This is a good idea whether or not you lease a space or work from home. To ensure profitability, your lease should not exceed 10 percent of this number.

Equipment

Purchase a reclining chair or massage table, rolling stool, shelving or cabinetry, desk, lighting, candles, a sound system and calming music, aromatherapy tools, linens, foot powder, foot and hand lotion, calming and cleaning products. You'll also need office supplies and accounting software that allows you to manage your clientele, schedule appointments, handle your inventory and expenses and calculate your taxes. As soon as possible, set up a merchant account at your bank to enable you to accept credit cards and hire an answering service to answer calls when you are busy with clients or record a message that tells clients that you can't answer the phone right now, however will get back to them as soon as possible. Don't go overboard in the beginning, purchase a few items at a time.

Policies

Establish a vision for your business and develop policies to help your clients have realistic expectations of your practice. While reflexology can minimize or treat a number of ailments, it won't necessarily happen overnight. Be sure to thoroughly explain the practice and benefits to avoid having clients hold too high an expectation. Also, be willing to pass those clients with severe conditions onto professionals skilled in those areas, such as physical or occupational therapists or yoga and clinical massage or other therapists.

Advertising

Refer back to those clients you met while volunteering your services and inform them that you have officially launched your practice. They should be more than happy to spread your name to friends and family. Get repeat clients by calling each client the day after the session to check up on their progress. Purchase a domain and set up your website. Start a reflexology blog. Establish relationships with others in the holistic field, such as yoga and Pilates instructors, health food store owners, osteopathic doctors, Chiropracters, physical therapists and nutritionists.

You may be able to set up a mutual advertising exchange system. Better yet, try to find a thriving Chiropractic parctice and if they don't already have a reflexologist on their staff, you might get to be the one. This way you get to work on the doctor's clientele and don't have to build up your own. They might even refer their client's too you. When you find an office to work out of, ask iof you can post your adverting out front to attract more people in. This way everyone wins.

Have your business cards printed early on and pass them out everywhere you go.

* * *

ABC's of Reflexology

Notes

Chapter XII

Pathology

(pă-thŏl'ə-jē) *n., pl.,* -gies.

1. The scientific study of the nature of disease and its causes, processes, development, and consequences. Also called *pathobiology.*

2. The anatomic or functional manifestations of a disease: *the pathology of cancer.*

3. A departure or deviation from a normal condition: *"Neighborhoods plagued by a self-perpetuating pathology of joblessness, welfare dependency, crime"* (Time).

(Peripheral) Neuropathy

The areas of the body most commonly affected by peripheral neuropathy are the feet and legs. Nerve damage in the feet can result in a loss of foot sensation, increasing the risk of foot problems. Injuries and sores on the feet may go unrecognized due to lack of sensation.

Therefore, you should learn proper skin and foot care. Rarely, other areas of the body such as the arms, abdomen, and back may be affected.

Symptoms of peripheral neuropathy may include:

- Tingling
- Numbness (severe or long-term numbness can become permanent)
- Burning (especially in the evening)
- Pain

In most cases, early symptoms of peripheral neuropathy will become less when blood sugar is under control. (*if the condition is caused by diabetes).

Plantar Fasciitis

Plantar Fasciitis is a painful inflammatory process of the plantar fascia. Long standing cases of plantar Fasciitis often demonstrate more degenerative changes than inflammatory changes, in which case they are termed plantar Fasciosis. The plantar fascia is a thick fibrous band of connective tissue originating on the bottom surface of the calcaneus (heel bone) and extending along the sole of the foot towards the five toes. It has been reported that plantar Fasciitis occurs in two million Americans a year and 10% of the population over a lifetime.

It is commonly associated with long periods of weight bearing. Among non-athletic populations, it is associated with a high body mass index.

The pain is usually felt on the underside of the heel and is often most intense with the first steps of the day. Another symptom is that the sufferer has difficulty bending the foot so that the toes are brought toward the shin (decreased dorsiflexion of the ankle). A symptom commonly recognized among sufferers of plantar Fasciitis is increased probability of knee pains, especially among runners.

Plantar Fasciitis is a common injury that can persist for years unless treatment is properly addressed. Plantar Fasciitis is an acute form of inflammation of the band of tissue running across the bottom of your foot.

Every time you flex your foot, those tendons, ligaments, and tissue move and when they are inflamed, every movement hurts. Once this tissue is injured it becomes very difficult to recover 100%.

It is almost impossible to keep from re-straining the area because even when the pain is gone you still aren't fully healed. But, when the pain disappears, that's when we start acting normally again even though your foot isn't fully healed.

It's just not possible to stop everything and rest the injury properly. Everyone has demands that make them keep going and when we are active we prevent the plantar from healing completely. We continually reinjure the area through our daily activities.

Bone Spurs

A bone spur (osteophyte) is a bony growth formed on normal bone. Most people think of something sharp when they think of a "spur," but a bone spur is just extra bone. It's usually smooth, but it can cause wear and tear or pain if it presses or rubs on other bones or soft tissues such as ligaments, tendons, or nerves in the body. Common places for bone spurs include the spine, shoulders, hands, hips, knees, and feet.

A bone spur forms as the body tries to repair itself by building extra bone. It generally forms in response to pressure, rubbing, or stress that continues over a long period of time.

Some bone spurs form as part of the aging process. As we age, the slippery tissue called cartilage that covers the ends of the bones within joints breaks down and eventually wears away (osteoarthritis). Also, the discs that provide cushioning between the bones of the spine may break down with age.

Over time, this leads to pain and swelling and, in some cases, bone spurs forming along the edges of the joint. Bone spurs due to aging are especially common in the joints of the spine and feet.

Bone spurs also form in the feet in response to tight ligaments, to activities such as dancing and running that put stress on the feet, and to pressure from being overweight or from poorly fitting shoes. For example, the long ligament on the bottom of the foot (plantar fascia) can become stressed or tight and pull on the heel, causing the ligament to become inflamed (plantar Fasciitis). As the bone tries to mend itself, a bone spur can form on the bottom of the heel (known as a "heel spur"). Pressure at the back of the heel from frequently wearing shoes that are too tight can cause a bone spur on the back of the heel. This is sometimes called a "pump bump," because it is often seen in women who wear high heels.

Bone spurs are usually caused by local inflammation, such as from degenerative arthritis or tendonitis. This inflammation stimulates the cells that form bone to deposit bone in this area, eventually leading to a bony prominence or spur. For example, inflammation of the ligament that surrounds a degenerating disc between the vertebrae (the bony building blocks of the spine) is a very common cause of bone spurs of the spine.

Inflammation of the Achilles tendon can lead to the formation of a bone spur at the back of the heel bone (calcaneus bone). This bone spur is sometimes referred to as a heel spur.

Neck and Back Pain Caused by Pronated Feet

Back and neck pain can have a wide variety of causes. Sometimes, the origin of the pain isn't the back and neck at all, but the feet.

Pronation is a term used to describe how the foot naturally rolls inward as a person walks or runs. With a normal foot, the heel strikes the ground, and the foot rolls inward through the progression of the step. Pronation is important because it absorbs shock. Some people, however, roll their feet too far inward, in a movement called overpronation. Overpronation often occurs in people with low arches or flat feet, and it can cause pain in multiple areas of the body.

Overpronation can cause a variety of injuries, especially in runners. The excessive turning of the foot can cause shin splints, plantar Fasciitis, bunions or Achilles tendonitis. Overpronation can also cause back and neck pain because the foot rolls too far inward, causing an ineffective gait that puts stress on the knees, hips, neck and back.

Tendonitis

A tendon is a tough yet flexible band of fibrous tissue. The tendon is the structure in your body that connects your muscles to the bones. The skeletal muscles in your body are responsible for moving your bones, thus enabling you to walk, jump, lift, and move in many ways. When a muscle contracts it pulls on a bone to cause movements. The structure that transmits the force of the muscle contraction to the bone is called a tendon.

Tendons come in many shapes and sizes. Some are very small, like the ones that cause movements of your fingers, and some are much larger, such as your Achilles tendon in your heel. When functioning normally, these tendons glide easily and smoothly as the muscle contracts.

Sometimes the tendons become inflamed for a variety of reasons, and the action of pulling the muscle becomes irritating. If the normal smooth gliding motion of your tendon is impaired, the tendon will become inflamed and movement will become painful. This is called **tendonitis**, and literally means inflammation of the tendon.

There are hundreds of tendons scattered throughout our body, but it tends to be a small handful of specific tendons that cause problems.

These tendons usually have an area of poor blood supply that leads to tissue damage and poor healing response.

This area of a tendon that is prone to injury is called a "watershed zone," an area when the blood supply to the tendon is weakest. In these watershed zones, they body has a hard time delivering oxygen and nutrients necessary for tendon healing--that's why we see common tendon problems in the same parts of the body.

Tendonitis is most often an overuse injury. Often people begin a new activity or exercise that causes the tendon to become irritated. Tendon problems are most common in the 40-60 year old age range. Tendons are not as elastic and forgiving as in younger individuals, yet bodies are still exerting with the same force.

Occasionally, there is an anatomical cause for tendonitis. If the tendon does not have a smooth path to glide along, it will be more likely to become irritated and inflamed. In these unusual situations, surgical treatment may be necessary to realign the tendon.

Arthritis

Arthritis of the feet is a disorder characterized by the swelling of the joints of the feet. Just like arthritis on other parts of the body, it can be painful and debilitating.

> Arthritis in general is one of the most common chronic infirmities in the United States, and affects about 350 million people in the world.

Types of Foot Arthritis

Osteoarthritis

Osteoarthritis can attack any of the 30 joints of the foot, but the big toe is more prone because it absorbs the most pressure during regular foot activities (such as walking). It also usually affects the ankle, the midfoot, and three joints of the hind foot. The cartilage erodes, causing the bone ends to fuse. This results stiffness and joint pains. Osteoarthritis results from wear and tear of cartilage in the feet. The cartilage of the joints become worn out over time, causing spurs (hardened areas) and subchondral cysts (pockets in the bone marrow filled with liquid). The bone deformation and the accumulation of the fluids cause the pain.

Rheumatoid arthritis

Rheumatoid arthritis is a systemic ailment, so it does not only affect the foot but also the entire body. It occurs when the internal parts of the foot's joints stiffen and swell. Rheumatoid arthritis causes the arch to collapse a little at a time, which causes the toes to contract and draw back. This condition is hereditary. Women are more prone to it. Rheumatoid arthritis is caused by an over active immune system.

The body's own immune cells attack it. There are a lot of different causes. In some persons, it is said, rheumatoid arthritis may be caused by genetic or hormonal factors.

Achilles Tendonitis

Achilles Tendonitis is a debilitating foot condition characterized by swelling of the Achilles tendon – the largest and strongest tendon in the body – more commonly known as the 'heel cord.' Athletes are especially prone to chronic Achilles Tendonitis. In fact, around 18% of serious runners experience it in their life.

If it is not treated properly, a simple Achilles Tendon injury can progress into Acute Achilles Tendonitis and make walking impossible.

Podiatrists recommend that the condition be treated as early as possible.

Achilles Tendonitis does not happen overnight, and usually does not manifest itself right away. Pain is usually mild at first, but it worsens with continued activity.

The first stage of the Achilles tendon injury, called Peritenonitis, has no visible symptoms. The patient may feel pain during activity or while at rest, but will not see any physical manifestation of damage.

As Achilles tendon injury progresses to the second stage (called Tendinosis), the patient may begin to notice some swelling or hard knots of tissue on the back of the leg.

If the feet are subjected to more physical activity and strain, the tendon may partially or completely rupture. This is the third stage (referred to as Peritenonitis with Tendinosis). The result is traumatic damage to the tendons – a condition that can prevent the legs from moving properly and require an extended recovery period.

Arch Pain (see Plantar Fasciitis)Arch pain, (also known as Tarsal Tunnel Syndrome) is the term used to describe the burning sensation under the long arches of the feet (arch strain).

This pain is caused by the swelling of the plantar arch, which is a group of mid-foot tissues that connects the toes to the heel bone. Arch pain also develops when the nerves at the ankle are pinched, causing pain to the arch (a condition known as tarsal tunnel syndrome).

The arch is a very important part of the foot. It facilitates the transfer of weight from the toes to the heel, among other things. When arch strain is severe, even the simplest foot movements can be extremely painful.

Morton's neuroma

Morton's neuroma refers to the enlargement of the nerve usually on the 3rd interspace – the nerve flanked by the third and fourth toes. This area is particularly prone because this is where a section of the lateral plantar nerve touches a section of the nerve of the medial plantar. Combined, these two nerves are usually larger (diameter-wise) than the nerves leading to the rest of the toes.

> There is still no consensus on why the nerve becomes enlarged to cause Morton's neuroma.

The nerve is also on the subcutaneous tissue, on top of the foot's fat pad near a vein and an artery. Right over the nerve is the deep transverse metatarsal ligament, which clutches the metatarsal bones and builds the nerve compartment's ceiling. As you walk, the ground shoves the inflamed nerve up, and the deep transverse metatarsal ligament shoves down, causing compression.

Patients suffering from Morton's neuroma usually experience pain (usually localized) in the 3rd and 4th toe interspace. For some patients, the pain is sharp, and for others it is dull. The pain is usually made worse by shoes and by walking, and is alleviated when the foot is not supporting any weight.

Flat feet seem to be a contributing factor. The nerve of a flat foot tends to abnormally pull in the direction of the middle, causing irritation and in some cases, nerve enlargement. Women seem to be more prone to Morton's neuroma, giving way to the theory that confining high-heeled shoes cause the condition. The heels and narrow toe boxes of women's shoes tend to transfer much of the body weight to the front part of the foot and compress toes, possibly squeezing the nerve section on all sides.

Morton's neuroma is diagnosed by palpating the area and pressing the toes from one side to another in order to elicit pain.

The reflologist may also press on the foot's affected interspace to stroke the neuroma. The reflexologist usually elicits Mulder's sign – an audible click when the reflexologist holds the patient's first three metatarsal heads with one hand and the last two metatarsal heads in the other and slightly pushes half of the foot up and half the foot down.

Callouses

Callouses (also called tyloma) develop when a certain area of the skin thickens to protect itself from repetitive friction or strain. Callouses are usually not painful, but are not pleasant to look at. When they do become painful, they need to be treated. Callus-prone areas include the feet, the hands, and other parts of the skin that are always rubbed or pressed. Foot calluses usually pop up on the plantar surface (more commonly known as the sole) and the metatarsals. Heel calluses can also appear on the heel. All these sections endure most of the pressure from daily activities such as standing and walking.

Blisters

Blisters are very common to athletes and people who wear socks everyday. They develop when socks stick to the sweaty skin of the feet. The rubbing that then takes place causes what is known as a blister.

When the feet and socks continue to rub against each other on the interior walls of the shoes, the outer layers of the feet's skin separate from their inner layers, and the space between these layers are filled with lymph fluid.

Blisters usually heal on their own. The blister fluid is reabsorbed and disappears. However, there are cases when the blisters pop (by themselves), causing them to become infected. Once redness, red lines, or yellow liquid develops around the blister, medical attention is required.

Three things cause foot blisters: moisture, heat and friction. Athletes, especially those who take part in very lengthy sporting events that require walking or running (such as marathons) – are prone to developing blisters.

New shoes that have not yet been broken in and other ill-fitting footwear tends to cause blisters, as well.

Blisters may also be caused by allergic reactions, fungal infections of the skin, burns, and excessive foot perspiration.

Metatarsalgia

Metatarsalgia denotes a foot condition characterized by pain and inflammation of the joints and bones of the ball of the foot – that area just before the toes, also called the metatarsal region. Most patients experience pain in the second, third and fourth metatarsal heads, but there are some cases of pain the big toe's metatarsal heads.

During walking, jumping, or running, a big percentage of your body weight transfers to the toes and therefore to the metatarsals. The metatarsal bones of the big toes together with the second and third metatarsals take the burden of weight transfer. Excessive pressure (common during athletic activities) sometimes leads to pain and swelling.

Metatarsalgia is not a very serious foot condition, but it can significantly affect foot movement. Athletes in high-impact sports such as basketball may find it very hard to jump and land because of Metatarsalgia, for example.

Fortunately, Metatarsalgia treatment is quite simple – in most cases, rest and some therapy are enough. Metatarsalgia surgery may be required with more severe cases.

Patients with Metatarsalgia usually experience a sharp, often 'burning' pain on the sole behind the toes, or 'balls' of the feet. The pain usually worsens when the patient stands, walks or runs or when the affected foot is flexed. The pain usually eases down with rest. Some patients also experience toe numbness. Most of these symptoms manifest abruptly, but it usually takes weeks for Metatarsalgia to develop.

One or a combination of many factors can cause Metatarsalgia.

Among the most common is over-training or over-activity. Studies show that runners – who tend to put excessive pressure on their metatarsals when playing – develop Metatarsalgia more than others do. Intensive, extended training puts an abnormal amount of stress on the balls of the feet, often causing irritation and eventually, inflammation.

A high arch, an abnormally long second toe, and other such structural factors can also cause Metatarsalgia. People with hammertoes, those who wear high heels (which prevent the toes from relaxing flat), and those who are overweight are also more prone to Metatarsalgia because their conditions tend to put more pressure on the balls of the feet.

The risk of developing Metatarsalgia also appears to go higher as a patient grown older. This is because the fat pads on the metatarsals thin out as a person ages, diminishing the ability of the metatarsal bones to protect themselves.

Sesamoiditis

Sesamoiditis refers to the irritation or inflammation of the tendons around the Sesamoids – bones in the feet that are embedded in the muscles or linked to the tendons (not to other bones). Sesamoids are located on the foot's outer side (near the middle area), and under the forefoot close to the big toe. These Sesamoids let tendons glide and manage transmission of the muscle's forces. They likewise elevate the bones of the big toe and help bear weight.

Sesamoiditis symptoms develop gradually. Patients usually feel slight aches that increase slowly and steadily until it becomes to feel like severe throbbing if he or she keeps on performing the triggering activity. Bruising or redness is usually not a symptom – in many cases, there is no other physical manifestation aside from swelling, which greatly affects dorsiflexion and plantar flexion (the capacity of the joint of the first metatarsophalangeal to bend upward and/or downward. The big toe cannot move, making walking very difficult.

Sesamoiditis is common among people who put a lot of stress on their Sesamoids, such as those in professions like ballet and those who engage in sports such as baseball (particularly baseball catchers and base runners).

Still, anyone can develop sesamoiditis, which is caused primarily by recurring, disproportionate pressure, tension, and stress on the forefoot, particularly on the first metatarsophalangeal joint. The tissues around the joint react to the tension by swelling up. People who frequently engage in activities that put constant stress on their feet's ball area can develop sesamoiditis. In fact, people who walk around constantly in unsupportive shoes can develop the condition.

Tarsal tunnel syndrome

Tarsal tunnel syndrome refers to the condition when the posterior tibial nerve is trapped in the tarsal tunnel – that space between the bones of the feet and corresponding tissue. It is compared to carpal tunnel syndrome (which happens on the wrist) because they are both triggered by the same cause – a nerve is pinched in a cramped area. The tarsal tunnel is very confined. Once it tightens, it pinches the tibial nerve. Tarsal Tunnel Syndrome and RSD have long been linked.

Reflex Sympathetic Dystrophy (RSD), which refers to recurring pain in the sympathetic nerve system because of triggers like trauma, injury, surgery, or infection, can occur alongside tarsal tunnel syndrome. In RSD, the trigger starts an irregular succession of pain (often intractable) and eventually set off total disability.

Most patients feel pain on the sole of the foot, often described as a burning or tingling sensation, because the nerves are compressed by entrapment. The pain is usually progressive. It becomes more severe into the day. Rest or elevation (sometimes even a massage) can help provide temporary relief.

Tarsal tunnel syndrome causes discomfort, sometimes even debilitation. And while it is more common in adults with very active lifestyles, children can develop it as well. The pain is caused by muscles adjacent to the tibial nerve that grow too big. They compact the tibial nerve, which then tries to send signals of pain to the brain. Its neurological impulses are limited, so it does not succeed and instead manifests in a burning or tingling sensation.

Flat-footedness can also cause tarsal tunnel syndrome. The flattened arches put pressure on the nerves and muscles surrounding the ankle, causing them to move way from their normal route, in turn, squeezing the tibial nerve.

Inflammation

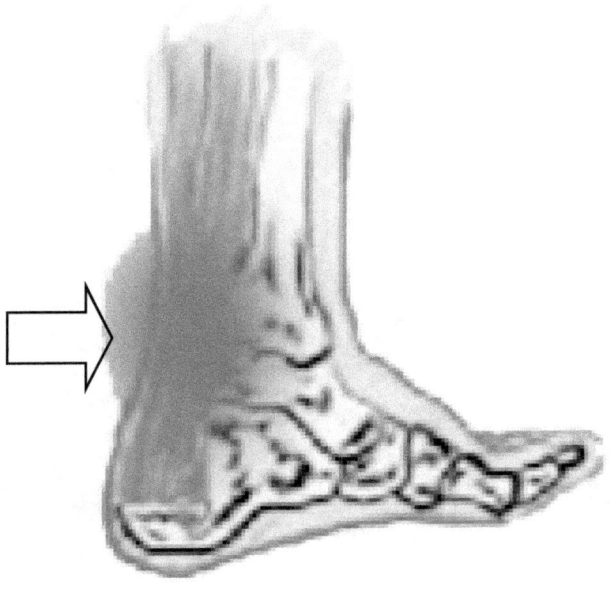

The arrow and picture above idicate an inflamed area of
irritation on the Achilles Tenden of the pictured foot.
Inflammation may occur in both or either left or right foot.

Plantar Fasciitis

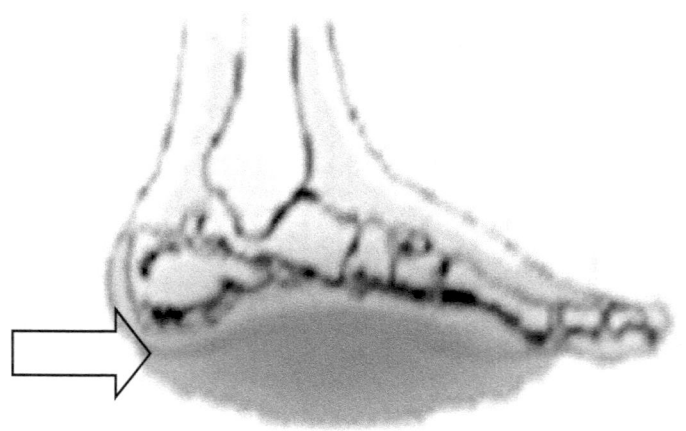

This is a very painful condition that makes walking and going anywhere extremely difficult. Plantar Fasciitis is very common in some age groups and can account for a large proportion of your regular clients.

Heel Spurs

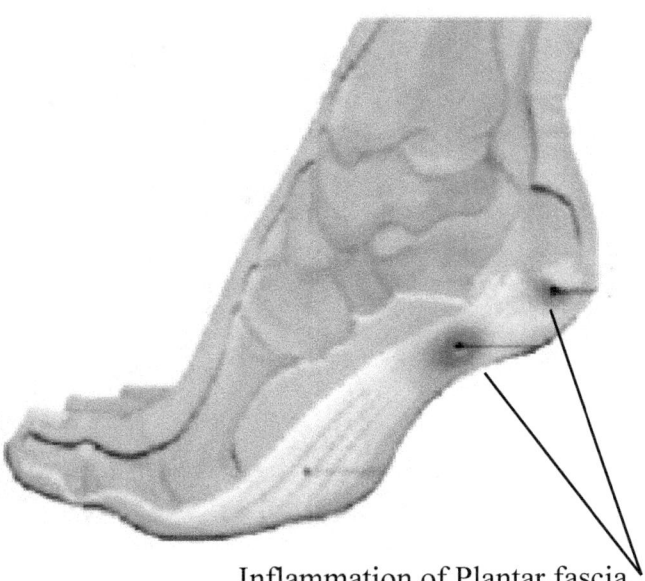

Inflammation of Plantar fascia

Two darker areas on heel indicate boney proturbances which press into fascia when walking. This again, can be very painful and limit mobility.

Arch Pain

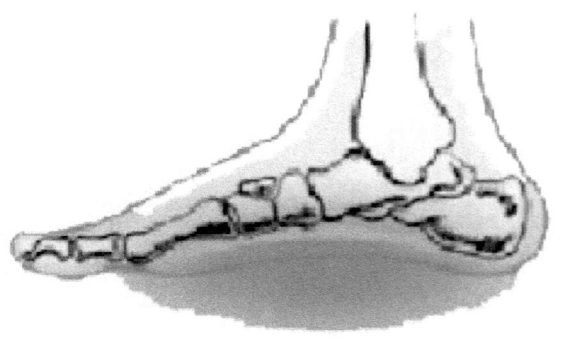

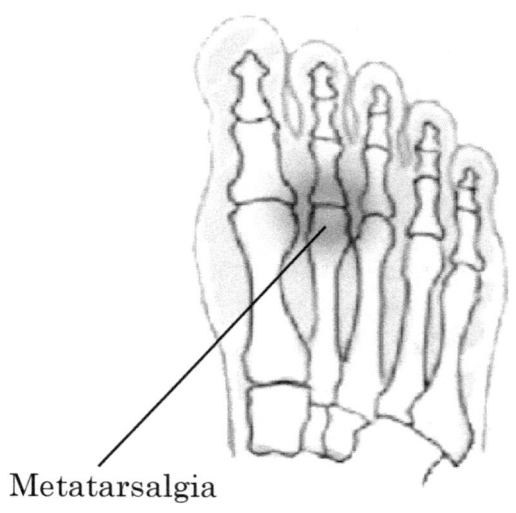

Metatarsalgia

Tarsal Tunnel Syndrome

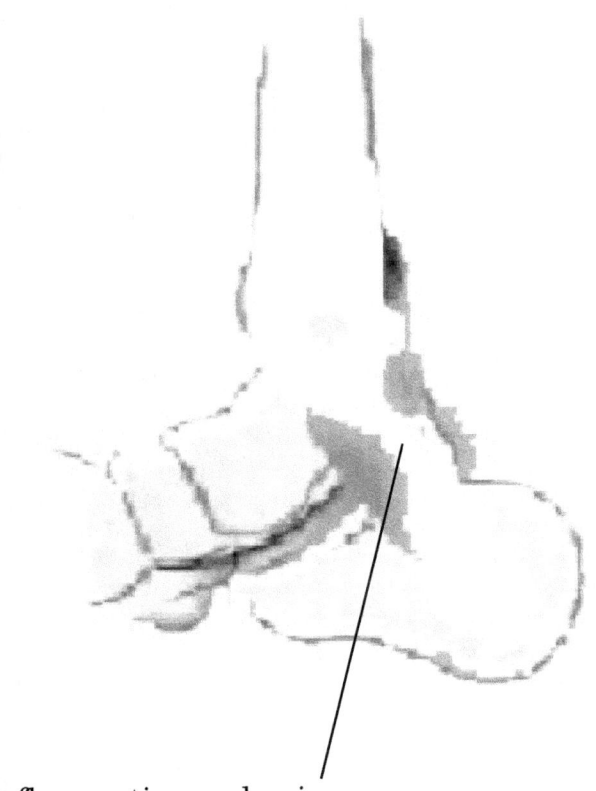

Inflammation and pain

Chapter XIII

Assessment

How to Read The Feet

Feet can tell you a lot about the body. Calluses, for instance, can tell you where there is stress in the body. Callus on the back of the heel tells you that you are pitching your weight to the lower back. Callus on the side of the big toe is a stress cue that could be pointing to stress at the base of the skull. Callus on the ball of the foot directly below the little toe could be pointing to shoulder pain.

Curled toes tell you a lot as well. They usually indicate hidden pain in the ball of the foot. The toes try to curl to protect the area and give you a little lift off the ground. It does not work very well but often points to tension in the upper back and chest. These are visual stress cues that are the easiest to pick out. But there are also touch and what we call "press and assess."

The later stress cue is fun in classes for picking out tailbone injuries. Bubbles will appear on the side of the foot when you press the heel. Always a crowd pleaser.

It's Important that the Client:

Understands reflexology is non-invasive. Inform them that at their appointments they will remain fully clothed except for socks and shoes. Have them sit or lie down as you wash their feet, wiping them with a gentle antiseptic and soaking them in warm water in preparation for the assessment.

Have them relax as you do an initial check of their feet for open wounds, rashes, sores, plantar warts or bunions. You should ask the client about their health, medical history, lifestyle, any foot or leg pain and the duration and intensity of any pain.

Have them breath normally as you explore by hand the soles of their feet for discomfort. Areas of concern indicate an imbalance and you will work those reflex areas to improve the function of the corresponding internal organs, glands, muscle groups, bones and nerves. At the end of the assessment, the client's feet should be moisturized and given a nice massage.

Prepare for your second appointment by asking the client for any signs of improvement to their health since the first visit.

Expect it to take 5 or 6 treatments before seeing significant improvement since nerve pathways and congestion must be worked on a bit to release toxins.

Assessment is the collection and interpretation of information provided by the Client, any referring health professionals and your own observation. Assessment requires methodically paying attention to what a client presents at this moment in time so that you can give appropriate and effective therapeutic action.

Assessment is NOT diagnosis.

The naming of a condition or problem is its diagnosis.

In the U.S., only physicians (MDs, DOs, NDs) and nurse practitioners (NPs) are licensed to give medical names (**medical diagnoses**) to diseases and illnesses, and this can vary from state to state. However, other health professionals also name (or diagnose) the health deviations they see according to their profession's established core philosophies, scope of practice, body of research and assessment, therapeutic action and outcome evaluation skills.

For instance, nurses make nursing diagnoses, licensed social workers and psychologists make psychological diagnoses and Traditional Chinese Medicine practitioners make TCM diagnoses. These types of diagnoses differ from medical ones in that they each use their own scope of practice, theories, body of research and therapeutic skill development to shape the language used. (Even auto mechanics "diagnose" our car problems.)

It is possible that when other body-centered professions develop their core theories, scope of practice, research base and assessment, therapeutic action and outcome evaluation skills further, then they will take up the task of developing their own system of diagnosis. In the mean time, it is important that we assess our clients by simply describing what we see, hear or feel.

The assessment process begins when you first see the client and is continual and on-going throughout each session. It culminates in a final assessment called an outcome evaluation near the end of the session. Assessments can be kept in your head if you never forget anything and can produce a printed copy of your assessment, two years later, upon request. (If you can do that, call us. We want to meet you.)

True assessment involves both art and science.

The science part involves applying your rational, structured knowledge about each client's anatomy, physiology and pathology to the work at hand. It requires you to know how each therapeutic action, or technique, you use effects the client, so that you can safely and effectively address his/her goals for the session. The art part involves applying your intuitive, artistic and creative abilities to synthesize the rational knowledge into a graceful, nurturing and effective experience for your client and yourself.

Each school, and probably each teacher, has his or her own style of assessment, based on personal philosophies, previous training and experience. However, the core components of an assessment are:

- client goal
- health history
- observation
- palpation

Assessment uses these components over and over again. Most of the process comes from a biomedical perspective because that is the perspective that is most widely available in the U.S. at this time, and it is the most thoroughly researched.

The Client's Goal

At the outset of each client's session with you, it is important to ask him or her: "What do you want from this work" The client's answer is the goal for the session. If the client answers "I don't know," it would be appropriate to clarify what information you are seeking. For instance, you can say that some people want to relax, some want to reduce pain and stiffness, some want to receive safe, nurturing touch, etc. This gives the client a place to start, and makes it easier to add their own personal feelings.

If a client wants something that you are not comfortable doing, it is important that you communicate this tactfully and immediately. Be congruent with your scope of practice, the *indications* and *contraindications* for your work, your education and your experience. For instance, perhaps a client asks you to "pop" her back, which is outside the scope of body-centered therapies unless you are a chiropractor. If you and the client are unable to reach a mutually comfortable understanding of the session's goal, then it is better for both of you to know that and deal with it in the beginning.

Remember that the client is the one paying for your service. If they don't feel better, they probably won't be back.

Health History

Each assessment begins with a review of the client's health history. A *health history* is a written record of past and current health events, including illnesses, accidents and surgeries. In the medical and psychiatric professions, the health history also includes major illnesses within the client's family, but most body-centered therapists do not need that information. If the client has consulted a physician or nurse practitioner for his or her current health problem, then the diagnosis of that problem can also be a helpful piece of information for you.

Most health histories are given by the client on his/her first visit, using a form that you provide. Many practitioners refer to this as an "intake form." It may include a statement of *consent* for the work. At the most primary level, a client is giving his or her "implied consent" for the work when she makes the appointment, shows up and follows whatever instructions the practitioner gives. In most cases of body-centered therapies, it would seem strange for the practitioner to ask the client to sign a consent form for the work, or ask the client "Is it OK if I touch you?" Permission is implied by the very nature of the relationship. However, in some cases, such as work with minors or other vulnerable persons, it is important to obtain written consent from a responsible

Federal laws require that health practitioners obtain written consent from their clients before they talk to or share records with any other health professional about that client. Any forms you choose to implement in your practice are legal documents. Please obtain legal advice before implementing any forms. If the client (or guardian) refuses to give you written consent to communicate with the attending physician or other health care team members when it is essential to the client's health or safety, then you should not treat the client.

Performing a health history on each client will help you in numerous ways: if done appropriately, the history process can show a client that you are willing to take the time and energy to get to know him / her - the process can give you information about who this person is and what has led him / her to this session; this makes your work more effective with less effort because you have information to guide your efforts the very act of writing about oneself helps the client be more consciously aware of his/her health; an increase in self-awareness can often facilitate an increase in self-responsibility during the history or intake process, you will often be able to sense which clients are expecting you to "fix" their problems, which is not your responsibility.

The sooner you realize that, the sooner you can enforce healthy boundaries for your work, saving yourself time, energy and frustration if your practice is ever reviewed in a court of law, having written records documents and limits your responsibility to the information you were given by the client.

There are several important questions to ask in a health history. The main questions are numbered, and the modifying questions, which can be either listed on a form or asked verbally, are indented with letters.

1) Have you ever received this type of work before?
 a) If so, were you sore (or other problem) afterwards?
2) What do you want from this work? (The answer becomes the client's goal for the session.)
3) Is there a current problem, pain or concern?
  a. If so, when did it start?
  b. If the problem involves pain, exactly where is it?
  c. What increases or decreases the problem?
  d. What have you been doing about the problem?
  e. What surgeries, illnesses or accidents might relate to the problem?
4) How do you spend most of your time? (Again, explore what might be contributing to the current problem.)

5) Do you exercise regularly?
   a) If so, how often and what do you do?

6) Are you under the care of another health practitioner? (The term "health practitioner" can include: MD, DO, chiropractor, nurse practitioner, social worker, psychologist, psychiatrist, dentist, podiatrist, herbalist, nutritionist, naturopath, shaman, etc.)

Some body-centered therapists have told us that assessments are not necessary in their practice because they only facilitate relaxation, comfort or nurturance. However, if they stop to think about it, they agree that they perform an informal assessment at the beginning, throughout the work and at the end of each session because they ask questions about what is going on with the client and they watch for changes that tell them the client is relaxing, feeling comforted and/or feeling nurtured.

If the client simply wants a simple relaxing session, has no ongoing problems or concerns, is not under a health practitioner's care and has no past history that would indicate either a particular benefit or caution, then the practitioner can proceed without any further questions. Otherwise, the questioning should continue and include:

If under another practitioner's care, what condition is being treated?

What is the therapy, medication or supplementation being used?

Use the answers to these questions, along with your training, experience and manual skills, to help you form the boundaries of your work with each person. Review the history/intake form prior to each session so that your memory about each person is refreshed. Ask the person if anything has changed since the last time you saw him/her, and if so add notes to update your information. Depending on your practice philosophy and style, there may be other questions you want to ask during the intake process and/or during the session. For more detailed information on health histories, see the Recommended Resources listed at the end of this course.

Observation and Palpation

Observation is looking and listening carefully with attention to detail. *Palpation* is the process of examining the foot (body) by applying one's hands to the foot or bodies surface. The process of observation and palpation is continuous, beginning when you first see the client and continuing throughout each session. Looking includes inspecting the client's posture, gait, behavior, breathing, skin tone, and range of motion. Pay particular attention to how the client talks, moves and breathes. Do these things suggest tension or stress? Relaxation? Function? Dysfunction?

Ease? Dis-ease? Patterns of asymmetry and movement can reveal important information about the body/mind, including muscular tension, soft tissue injury and/or dysfunction.

Listening includes hearing both what is said to you and how it is said. It includes asking respectful, attentive questions before, during and after the work and waiting to hear the answers. Open-ended questions encourage more sharing of information. For example, the question "Have you ever had this type of work?" only asks for a "yes" or "no" answer. The question "What is your experience with body centered therapies?" invites a much more informative answer.

Feeling includes physical *palpation* of the client's feet and legs, feeling for lumps, tightness, looseness, springiness, etc. The word palpation means the process of examining by touch. Palpation,like assessment, is an art and a science. Palpation is used extensively in Massage Therapy but is just as relevant to the Reflexologist. Body therapists perform physical palpation more than any other health professional. If you can use your hands to gather information, process it through your body-mind and make treatment choices that benefit the client, it is a remarkable and wonderful gift, Feeling also includes intuitive feeling, in whatever ways that happen for you.

Pay particular attention to what you feel (remember the chapter on intuition?), and keep learning.

* * *

Additional Resources

Acupressure and Reflexology For Dummies by Bobbi Dempsey and Synthia Andrews, Sep 4, 2007.

Body Reflexology: Healing at Your Fingertips by Mildred Carter and Tammy Weber ,Jul 15, 2002.

Complete Reflexology for Life by Barbara Kunz, Aug 17, 2009.

Hands On Feet The New System That Makes Reflexology a Snap by Michelle R. Kluck Jul 10, 2001.

Reflexology: Therapeutic Foot Massage for Health and Well-being (Complete Illustrated Guide) by Inge Dougans and Paul Allen, Aug 5, 1999.

The Reflexology Atlas by Bernard C. Kolster M.D. and Astrid Waskowiak M.D., Jan 9, 2006.

The Reflexology Manual: An Easy-to-Use Illustrated Guide to the Healing Zones of the Hands and Feet by Pauline Wills, Oct 1, 1995.

The Joy of Reflexology: Healing Techniques for the Hands and Feet to Reduce Stress and Reclaim Life by Ann Gillanders, Mar 1, 1996.

The Complete Reflexology Tutor: Everything You Need to Achieve Professional Expertise by Ann Gillanders , Jan 1, 2008.

Reflexology: A Basic Guide by Beryl Crane, Metro Books, 1999.

Reflexology with Michelle Kluck, Living Arts VHS Cassette, MXCIX

Simply Reflexology (DVD), 2006, Hinkler Books. Australia.

* * *

Conditions and Treatment

Condition	Reflex Areas
Acne	Solar plexus / diaphragm, chest / lung, thyroid and helper to thyroid, pituitary, intestines, kidneys, adrenals, liver
Adenoid Problems	Solar plexus / diaphragm, chest / lung, bronchials, sinuses, pituitary
Alcoholism	Solar plexus / diaphragm, chest / lung, bronchials, heart, brain, pineal, pituitary, hypothalamus, pancreas, liver, bladder, ureters, kidneys
Allergies	Solar plexus / diaphragm, chest / lung, thyroid and helper to thyroid, all toes with emphasis on pituitary, sinuses ileocecal valve, intestines, adrenals Breast / chest, lymph neck / chest, thymus, big toes with emphasis on throat and nose, reproductive glands, chronic reproductive, lymph / groin
Anemia	Thyroid and helper to thyroid, heart, spleen, liver
Angina Pectoris	Solar plexus / diaphragm, chest / lung, heart, shoulder / arm, neck, thoracic and cervical spine, intestines with emphasis on sigmoid colon, duodenum, adrenals
Appendicitis	Solar plexus / diaphragm, appendix / ileocecal valve, intestines, duodenum, adrenals
Arthritis	Entire foot with emphasis on the following: spine, parathyroids, solar plexus / diaphragm, kidneys, adrenals, reflex for afflicted area
Asthma	Solar plexus / diaphragm, chest / lung, shoulder / arm, bronchials, heart, sinuses, ileocecal valve, intestines, adrenals Breast / chest, shoulder / arm, reproductive glands, chronic reproductive
Back Problems	Solar plexus / diaphragm, spine, shoulder / arm, neck, sciatic Spine, neck, shoulder / arm, mid-back, sciatic, hip / sciatic, leg, knee
(Upper Back)	Solar plexus / diaphragm, spine with emphasis on cervical and thoracic spine, shoulder / arm, neck, sciatic
(Lower Back)	Spine, with emphasis on lumbar, sacral, coccyx, solar plexus / diaphragm, sciatic
Bed Wetting	Solar plexus / diaphragm, spine with emphasis on lumbar, brain, bladder, ureters, kidneys, adrenals
Bladder Problems	Solar plexus / diaphragm, chest / lung, bronchials, lower spine with emphasis on lumbar, bladder, ureters, kidneys, adrenals

Breast (lumps)	Solar plexus / diaphragm, chest / lung, heart, shoulder / arm, thoracic spine with emphasis on T1-7, pituitary, bladder, ureters, kidneys Breast / chest, lymph neck / chest, thymus, mid-back, thoracic spine, bladder
Bronchitis	Solar plexus / diaphragm, chest / lung, bronchials, heart, shoulder / arm, thoracic spine with emphasis on T1-7, ileocecal valve, intestines, adrenals Breast / chest, lymph neck / chest, shoulder / arm, thoracic spine, mid-back
Bursitis	Solar plexus / diaphragm, chest / lung, shoulder / arm, spine, kidneys, adrenals, sciatic, referral area to afflicted part of body Breast / chest, lymph neck / chest, shoulder / arm, spine, mid-back, knee / leg / hip, hip / sciatic, sciatic, lymph / groin, thymus
Calluses (Bunions)	Work directly on and around the affected area
Cataracts	Eye / ear / neck, cervicals, all toes with emphasis on pituitary, thyroid and helper to thyroid, kidneys
Cholesterol	Solar plexus / diaphragm, thyroid and helper to thyroid, heart, liver, gall bladder
Cirrhosis of the Liver	
Colds	Solar plexus / diaphragm, chest / lung, bronchials, thyroid and helper to thyroid, shoulder / arm, eye / ear / neck, esophagus, all toes with emphasis on pituitary, stomach, spleen, ileocecal valve, intestines, duodenum, adrenals, liver Breast / chest, lymph, neck / chest, inner ear, thymus, shoulder / arm, all toes with emphasis on throat and nose
Colitis	Solar plexus / diaphragm, intestines, duodenum, adrenals, liver, gallbladder, lower spine Lymph / groin
Conjunctivitis	(see Eye Disorders)
Constipation	Solar plexus / diaphragm, lower spine, spleen, ileocecal valve, intestines, duodenum, adrenals, liver, gallbladder, sciatic Lower spine, sciatic, hip / sciatic, hip / knee / leg
Corns	(see Calluses)
Cystitis	Lower spine, bladder, ureters, kidneys, adrenals Lower spine, lymph / groin, hip / sciatic, hip / knee, bladder
Depression	Solar plexus / diaphragm, chest / lung, shoulder /arm, neck, heart, thyroid and helper to thyroid, parathyroids, all toes with emphasis on pituitary brain, pancreas, adrenals Breast / chest, thymus, shoulder / arm, neck / throat

* These numbers refer to pages in the original manual.

Diabetes	Solar plexus / diaphragm, thyroid and helper to thyroid, heart, pituitary, pancreas, liver, adrenals
Diarrhea	Solar plexus / diaphragm, lower spine, ileocecal valve, intestines, duodenum, adrenals, lower Lower spine, chronic rectal
Disc Problems	Solar plexus / diaphragm, spine with emphasis on affected area, neck, shoulder / arm, brain, sciatic Spine, neck / throat, shoulder / arm, mid back, sciatic, hip / sciatic
Diverticulitis	Solar plexus / diaphragm, lower spine intestines with emphasis on sigmoid colon, duodenum, adrenals, liver, gallbladder
Dizziness	Solar plexus / diaphragm, all toes with emphasis on pituitary, cervicals, helper to eye / ear, inner ear, cervicals
Earache	Solar plexus / diaphragm, all toes, cervicals, helper to eye / ear, adrenals Thymus, lymph, neck / chest, inner ear, neck / throat, upper and lower jaw, cervicals
Eczema	Solar plexus / diaphragm, chest / lung, thyroid and helper to thyroid, pituitary, intestines, kidneys, duodenum, adrenals, pancreas, lower Breast / chest, lymph, neck / chest, thymus, lymph / groin
Edema	Solar plexus / diaphragm, heart, bladder, ureters, kidneys, adrenals, reflex and referral for afflicted area Lymph neck / chest, lymph / groin, bladder
Emphysema	Solar plexus / diaphragm, chest / lung, bronchials, neck, cervical and thoracic spine, ileocecal valve, intestines, adrenals Breast / chest, lymph, neck / chest, throat, nose, cervicals, thoracic spine, mid-back
Epilepsy	Solar plexus / diaphragm, spine, neck, throat, thyroid and helper to thyroid, all toes with emphasis on brain and pituitary, pancreas, ileocecal valve, intestines, adrenals
Eye, Neck & Shoulder Strain	
Eye Disorders	Helper to eye / ear, all toes with emphasis on brain, cervicals, kidneys
Fainting	Heart, all toes with emphasis on pituitary and brain, cervicals
Fatigue	Solar plexus / diaphragm, heart, thyroid and helper to thyroid, spine, all toes with emphasis on pituitary and brain, spleen, pancreas, liver, adrenals

ABC's of Reflexology

Fever	Thyroid and helper to thyroid, all toes with emphasis on brain, pituitary and hypothalamus, cervicals, kidneys, spleen, ureters, bladder, and liver Lymph, neck / chest, thymus, cervicals, lymph / groin
Flatulence	Solar plexus / diaphragm, esophagus, lower spine, intestines with emphasis on sigmoid colon, duodenum, stomach, pancreas, liver, gallbladder
Fracture	Corresponding part of foot, referral areas
Gallstones	Solar plexus / diaphragm, thyroid and helper to thyroid, thoracic spine, liver, gallbladder
Gas Pains	(see Flatulence)
Glaucoma	Solar plexus / diaphragm, helper to eye / ear, all toes with emphasis on pituitary, cervicals, kidneys
Gout	Solar plexus / diaphragm, lover, kidneys, referral and reflex for afflicted area Lymph neck / chest, lymph / groin
Growths, Abnormal	Referral and reflex for afflicted area, pituitary, spleen
Halitosis	Solar plexus / diaphragm, esophagus, stomach, duodenum, lover, intestines, all toes Teeth, gums / upper jaw, teeth, gums / lower jaw
Hay Fever	Solar plexus / diaphragm, chest / lung, bronchials, cervicals, neck, all toes with emphasis on sinuses and pituitary, eyes, ileocecal valve, intestines, adrenals Breast / chest, lymph, neck / chest, thymus, throat / neck and nose, cervicals, lymph / groin, reproductive glands, chronic reproductive
Headache	Solar plexus / diaphragm, shoulder / arm, neck, thyroid and helper to thyroid, spine with emphasis on cervicals, all toes with emphasis on pituitary, brain and sinuses, pancreas, ileocecal valve, intestines and adrenals, sciatic Spine, thymus, lymph, neck / chest, neck / throat, upper and lower jaw, mid back, reproductive glands, chronic reproductive, sciatic, hip / sciatic, breast / chest and shoulder / arm
Hearing Problems	Shoulder / arm, eye / ear / neck, all toes with emphasis on brain, pituitary and sinuses, cervicals
Heart Attack	Solar plexus / diaphragm, chest / lung, heart, shoulder / arm, spine with emphasis on thoracic spine, brain, pituitary, intestines with emphasis on sigmoid colon, kidneys, adrenals
Heartburn	Solar plexus / diaphragm, chest / lung, heart, esophagus, thoracic spine, intestines, duodenum, pancreas, stomach, gallbladder

Hemorrhoids	Solar plexus / diaphragm, heart, lumbar, coccyx, sacral, intestines with emphasis on sigmoid colon, adrenals, sciatic Sciatic, chronic rectum, hip / sciatic, hip / knee / leg, lower spine
Hernia	Solar plexus / diaphragm, lower spine, intestines, adrenals Lower spine, hip / sciatic, hip / knee, lymph / groin
Hiatal Hernia	Solar plexus / diaphragm, chest / lung, esophagus, thoracic spine, stomach, adrenals
Hiccoughs	Solar plexus / diaphragm, chest / lung, heart, esophagus, bronchials, shoulder / arm, thoracic spine, neck, toes, stomach
High Blood Pressure	Solar plexus / diaphragm, chest / lung, spine, heart, thyroid, and helper to thyroid, pituitary, kidneys, adrenals
Hip Problems	Solar plexus / diaphragm, shoulder, lower back with emphasis on sacral, sciatic Lower back, sciatic, hip / sciatic, hip / knee, shoulder, lymph / groin
Hot Flashes	(see Menopause)
Hyperactivity	Solar plexus / diaphragm, thyroid, and helper to thyroid, brain, pituitary, adrenals, pancreas, liver
Hypoglycemia	Thyroid and helper to thyroid, pituitary, pancreas, liver, kidneys, adrenals
Hysterectomy	Solar plexus / diaphragm, thyroid and helper to thyroid pituitary, lower back, sciatic, adrenals Chronic reproductive, lower back, sciatic, hip / sciatic, reproductive glands, fallopian tubes, lymph / groin, hip / knee, thymus
Impotence	Solar plexus / diaphragm, chest / lung, thyroid and helper to thyroid, brain, pituitary, lower spine, pancreas and adrenals Breast / chest, thymus, lower back, chronic reproductive, reproductive glands, penis, seminal vesicles, hip / sciatic, hip / knee
Incontinence	Solar plexus / diaphragm, lower back, bladder, ureters, kidneys, adrenals
Indigestion	Solar plexus / diaphragm, thoracic and lumbar spine, esophagus, stomach, pancreas, liver, gallbladder, duodenum intestines Gums, teeth, neck / throat, lower spine
Infections	Adrenals, tonsils, thymus, spleen Thymus, lymph neck / chest, lymph / groin, reflex to afflicted area
Infertility	Solar plexus / diaphragm, thyroid and helper to brain, pituitary, lower back, adrenals Chronic reproductive, reproductive glands, fallopian tubes / seminal vesicles, lower back

Influenza	Solar plexus / diaphragm, chest / lung, bronchials, thyroid and helper to thyroid, all toes with emphasis on pituitary, intestines, adrenals Breast / chest, lymph, neck / chest, thymus, lymph / groin
Insomnia	Solar plexus / diaphragm, chest / lung, shoulder, neck, thyroid and helper to thyroid, all toes with emphasis on brain, pineal and pituitary, pancreas, adenoids
Jaundice	Thoracic spine, liver, gallbladder
Kidney Problems	Solar plexus / diaphragm, lower back, bladder, ureters, kidneys, adrenals
Kidney Stones	Solar plexus / diaphragm, parathyroid, lower back, bladder, ureters, kidneys, adrenals
Knee Problems	Spine, shoulder, sciatic, referral area is elbow Spine, sciatic, hip / sciatic, knee / leg / hip, mid-back, shoulder
Laryngitis	Solar plexus / diaphragm, chest / lung, neck, all toes cervicals, adrenals Breast / chest, lymph, neck / chest, vocal cords, neck / throat
Leg Problems	Spine, shoulder, kidneys, adrenals, sciatic, referral for afflicted area Spine, sciatic, hip / sciatic, knee / leg / hip, lymph / groin, mid-back, shoulder
Liver Conditions	Solar plexus / diaphragm, chest / lung, heart, thoracic spine, liver, gallbladder
Low Blood Pressure	Solar plexus / diaphragm, chest / lung, heart, thyroid and helper to thyroid, parathyroids, pituitary, kidneys, adrenals
Menopause	Solar plexus / diaphragm, thyroid and helper to thyroid, parathyroids, brain, pituitary, kidneys, adrenals Chronic reproductive, reproductive glands, fallopian tube, hip / sciatic, hip / knee
Menstrual Problems	Solar plexus / diaphragm, chest / lung, thyroid and helper to thyroid, parathyroids, brain, pituitary, pancreas, adrenals, lower back Breast / chest, lymph, neck / chest, thymus, lower back, chronic reproductive, reproductive glands, hip / sciatic, hip / knee, lymph / groin
Migraine	(see Headache)
Morning Sickness	Solar plexus / diaphragm, thyroid and helper to thyroid, pituitary, stomach, adrenals Chronic reproductive, reproductive glands
Motion Sickness	Solar plexus / diaphragm, spine, helper to eye / ear, brain, pituitary, stomach Spine, inner ear, mid-back

Nausea	Solar plexus / diaphragm, chest / lung, thyroid and helper to thyroid, esophagus, pituitary, stomach, liver, gallbladder, adrenals
Neck Problems	Solar plexus / diaphragm, shoulder, neck, spine with emphasis on cervicals, all toes, adrenals
Nervousness	Solar plexus / diaphragm, thyroid and helper to thyroid, spine, brain, pituitary, adrenals, pancreas
Numbness in Fingertips	Solar plexus / diaphragm, shoulder / arm, heart, spine with emphasis on seventh cervical, referral area is all toes
Paralysis	Entire foot with emphasis on solar plexus / diaphragm, spine, neck and brain, reflex for afflicted area
Perspiring Hands/Feet	Solar plexus / diaphragm, thyroid and helper to thyroid, pituitary, liver, intestines, kidneys, adrenals
Phlebitis	Solar plexus / diaphragm, heart, liver, intestines, adrenals, sciatic; referral area is arm Sciatic, hip / sciatic, knee / leg / hip, lymph / groin, thymus
Pneumonia	Solar plexus / diaphragm, chest / lung, shoulder / arm, neck, thyroid and helper to thyroid, thoracic spine, intestines, adrenals, pituitary, eye / ear Breast / chest, shoulder / arm, lymph neck / chest, thymus, thoracic spine, neck / throat
Pregnancy	Solar plexus / diaphragm, thyroid and helper to thyroid, spine, pituitary, sciatic, bladder, adrenals Breast / chest, thymus, lymph neck / chest, mid-back, spine, sciatic, chronic reproductive, reproductive glands, vagina, fallopian tubes, hip / sciatic, knee / leg / hip, bladder
Prostate Problems	Solar plexus / diaphragm, pituitary, lower back, bladder, adrenals, sciatic Lower back, sciatic, chronic reproductive, reproductive glands, seminal vesicles, lymph / groin, bladder
Psoriasis	Solar plexus / diaphragm, chest / lung, thyroid and helper to thyroid, pituitary, intestines, kidneys, adrenals, liver
Rheumatism	(see Arthritis and Bursitis)
Sciatica	Solar plexus / diaphragm, shoulder, spine, sciatic Shoulder / arm, sciatic, hip / sciatic, knee / leg / hip, lymph / groin, spine, mid-back
Scoliosis	Solar plexus / diaphragm, chest / lung, shoulder / arm, neck, thyroid and helper to thyroid, spine, pituitary, adrenals
Shingles	Solar plexus / diaphragm, chest / lung, shoulder / arm, neck, thyroid and helper to thyroid, spine, pituitary, adrenals Breast / chest, lymph, neck / chest, shoulder / arm, thymus, neck / throat, spine, lymph / groin

Shoulder Pains	Solar plexus / diaphragm, chest / lung, shoulder / arm, neck, spine with emphasis on upper back Breast / chest, lymph, neck / chest, shoulder / arm, mid-back, hip / sciatic, hip / knee, spine
Sinusitis	Solar plexus / diaphragm, chest / lung, bronchials, neck, all toes with emphasis on sinuses and pituitary, cervicals, ileocecal valve, intestines, adrenals
Skin Disorders	Solar plexus / diaphragm, , thyroid and helper to thyroid, pituitary, intestines, kidneys, adrenals Reproductive glands
Sore Throat	Solar plexus / diaphragm, neck, all toes, cervicals, adrenals Lymph neck / chest, thymus, cervicals, neck / throat
Sprain	Solar plexus / diaphragm, chest / lung, heart, adrenals, reflex for afflicted area Breast / chest, lymph neck / chest, lymph / groin
Spur on Heel	
Stroke	Solar plexus / diaphragm, heart, spine, all toes with emphasis on brain (opposite side from the paralysis), reflex for afflicted area
Teeth and Gum Disorders	All toes, cervicals Lymph neck / chest, neck / throat, teeth / gums upper jaw, teeth / gums lower jaw
Tinnitus	Solar plexus / diaphragm, eye / ear / neck, all toes, cervicals, adrenals
Tonsillitis	Solar plexus / diaphragm, eye /e ear / neck, all toes, cervicals, adrenals Lymph neck / chest, thymus, cervicals, neck / throat
Tumors	Thyroid and helper to thyroid, pituitary, adrenals, reflex for afflicted area
Ulcer	Solar plexus / diaphragm, chest / lung, heart, esophagus, , thyroid and helper to thyroid, neck, thoracic and lumbar spine, stomach, intestines, duodenum, adrenals Breast / chest, lymph neck / chest, thymus, thoracic and lumbar spine, lymph / groin, mid-back
Varicose Veins	Solar plexus / diaphragm, chest / lung, heart, , thyroid and helper to thyroid, pituitary, liver, intestines, adrenals, reflex for afflicted area
Vertigo	(see Dizziness)
Vitality Loss	Solar plexus / diaphragm, , thyroid and helper to thyroid, spine, brain, pituitary, adrenals, pancreas
Whiplash	Solar plexus / diaphragm, chest / lung, shoulder / arm, neck, spine with emphasis on cervicals, adrenals Breast / chest, lymph neck / chest, neck / throat, shoulder, spine, mid-back

About The Authors

Benita Babeckis: is a certified Hypnotherapist and Reflexologist with a Doctorate in Theology. She is also a Reiki Master, Karuna Master and an NLP Master & Trainer. Benita is NTCB certified in Reflexology as an instructor and has been a practioner for fourteen years.

Jim Babeckis: is a Massage Therapist, Craniosacral Therapist, a Certified Reiki Master, and an NLP Master & Trainer. Jim has a Doctorate in Theology and both a BA and MA in Psychology earned while in his 60's.

Together: they have been keynote speakers at the Mid-America Hypnosis Conference. They have taught Psychic Development classes and published "On Gossamer Wings" Springfield Illinois' only locally owned New Age Newsletter. After moving to Tucson they formed Tranzformations, continue to teach and have written more than twenty-five books, workbooks and reports. They have successfully started, managed and run businesses in several locations in Illinois, as well as in Tucson. They have written some fifteen books.

Other Books By Benita And Jim

Renewal

Feeling stressed? Anxious? Nervous? Learn what behaviors can feed stress and how to change these behaviors to reduce it. Learn stress management and the best ways to deal with panic attacks. Find other resources to help you cope with anxiety.
ISBN # 978-1440413347

Put Your Weight Loss in Overdrive

Do you want to lose weight? Are you willing to eat healthier and make changes in your diet? If you are willing to follow our lead and replace your unhealthy diet with even some of the super foods we tell you about in this book, you will put your diet in overdrive. Weight loss will be a snap. We guarantee it. This book makes weight loss easy.   ISBN # 978-1440413320

Life Management

Are you organized? Then you aren't the person we're looking for. If you aren't as organized as you think you should be, this is the book for you. Say goodbye to clutter and let order reign. We provide clever home and family management tips.; time saving tips and more. Get help managing your life.   ISBN # 978-1440417458

You Want It When?
Are you a procrastinator? Do you put off doing things until just before they're due? Do you do your Christmas shopping on Christmas Eve? There is help for all of you right here. Learn how to break the procrastination habit. ISBN # 978-1440417067

ABC's of Goal Setting
Ever set goals and write them down? What happened? Did you reach any of them or did you give up before you got there? Supercharge your goal setting and get ready for that satisfaction that only comes after reaching one of your goals. This book makes goal setting easy. ISBN # 978-1440419183

How Toxic Are You?
Everyone is subjected to toxins everyday. Over 80,000 at last count. Living away from the larger cities helps but not as much as you think. There are toxins in our water, our food, and in our air. What can we do to be healthy and survive our toxic world? Does fasting or jogging help? Yes, but not enough – toxins bind to fat cells. If you are at all interesting in your and your families health, this is a must read! ISBN # 978-140425590

The Family Book of Fairy Tales
Stories of Princes and Princess's, enchanted giants and mighty ogres, lions, tailors and onions collected from around the world and assembled in this book to amuse you and your children. Includes the following stories: Cinderella's Daughter, The Giant's Hand, The Prince and the Lions, The Three Buns, The Boyer's Bride, How the Sea Became Salt, The Captive Princess, The Enchanted Oranges, The Knight of the Onion Shield, The Trade That No One Knew and The Prince and The Tailor. ISBN # 978-1441435057

Coming Soon!

The Castle of the Grail
The Quest for the Grail is not a fairy tale for children. It is a serious undertaking. The journey is full of trials and tribulations. The inner landscape of the Quest is full of dark forests, winding paths, narrow places, bridges, gates and castles. It is a very confusing place for us because we start foolish and ignorant. We do not recognize our guide and are frightened of what we might find. We are tested severely and ruthlessly but with mercy. The Quest is about Self Transformation and personal liberation. There is a unifying principle at the heart of all of these ways of thought, which can only be grasped by symbols, analogies and myths. Jung explained this with his archetypes of the collective unconscious.
ISBN # (not yet assigned)

The Gold Mine in PLR.
What is PLR? How can it benefit you? P.L. and R. are the initial letters of Private Label Rights. PLR is merchandise or software, most of which is info or text based, customizable, and reusable as your own. The concept of PLR differs only slightly from having a ghostwriter. So if you have a website and need fresh content or are a writer and need fresh ideas - this book is a must have! ISBN # (not yet assigned)

Creativity
Would you like to be more creative? More intuitive? Would you like to learn creative problem solving? You can with the proper training. You probably already are intuitive and creative without realizing it. This book will provide the training you need to handle anything life throws at you in a more creative way. ISBN # (not yet assigned)

Take Control (It's Your Book)
Covers everything the author needs to know about self publishing. Copyrights, ISBN numbers, writing software versus page layout software, cover design, book layout, POD versus conventional printing methods, marketing, distribution, advertising, etc. ISBN # (not yet assigned)

Benita's Encyclopedia of Crystals and Stones
What gems, crystals or stones have healing properties? Which do not? Which stones would you use for High Blood Pressure? Which for blood disorders? Which stones would be more effective for sores and wounds? How would you use Calcite in healing? ISBN # (not yet assigned)

Handy Order Form

Telephone orders: 520-609-9135 Have your credit card handy.

Email orders: Tranzform@Comcast.net <Attn. Orders>

Postal orders: Orders * 8571 N. Calle Tioga * Oro Valley, Az. 85704

Please send the following books, software or reports. I understand that I may return any of them for a full refund for any reason.

ISBN No. _____ Quantity ☐

Title: _____

ISBN No. _____ Quantity ☐

Title: _____

Name: _____

Address: _____

City:_____ State:_____ Zip:_____

Phone: _____

Email: _____

I would like more information on other books and/ or products -------------------------------- ☐

Arizona residents please add 8.1% Sales tax.